ELECTROTHERAPY AND ACTINOTHERAPY

CLAYTON'S
Electrotherapy
and
Actinotherapy

A TEXTBOOK FOR
STUDENT PHYSIOTHERAPISTS

Pauline M. Scott

M.C.S.P., Dip. T.P.
School of Physiotherapy
King's College Hospital, London

SIXTH EDITION

Baillière Tindall & Cassell
LONDON

First published 1948
Second edition 1951
Third edition 1959
Fourth edition 1962
Fifth edition 1965
Sixth edition 1969

© *Baillière Tindall and Cassell Ltd.*, 1969
7–8 Henrietta Street, London, WC2

7020 0312 3

*Published in the United States by
the Williams & Wilkins Company, Baltimore*

Printed in Great Britain

PREFACE TO THE SIXTH EDITION

THIS book is intended primarily for the use of physiotherapy students, being designed to cover the electrotherapy sections of the syllabus for the examinations of the Chartered Society of Physiotherapy. As far as possible the work is confined to basic principles and aims at stressing those points which are of importance to the physiotherapist.

The principal changes in this edition are that a chapter on microwave diathermy has been added and the one on ultrasonic therapy amplified. The chapters on the constant D.C. and ionisation have been deleted, together with some other obsolete items. The circuits of modern short-wave diathermic machines, formerly included in the section on interference with radio reception, have been omitted. These circuits never formed part of the syllabus for the C.S.P. examinations, and continual developments make it difficult to keep the accounts up to date. Certain other additions and deletions have been made, in an attempt to keep abreast of modern thought and methods.

I have often received enquiries regarding the origin of this book. Dr. E. Bellis Clayton was director of the Department of Physical Medicine at King's College Hospital from 1912 until his retirement in 1946. The School of Physiotherapy was opened in 1915, and Dr. Clayton worked untiringly for the furtherance of physiotherapy and the welfare of the staff and students, by whom he was much beloved. He taught much of the light and diathermy and had notes of his lectures printed for the use of the students. These formed the basis of his book *Actinotherapy and Diathermy* which was published in 1939, and was followed in 1944 by *Electrotherapy*, dealing with the direct and low frequency currents. In 1948 the two books were amalgamated into *Electrotherapy and Actinotherapy* and when, in 1958, Dr. Clayton felt unable to produce a further edition, I was honoured to be entrusted with its preparation. As I already owe much to Dr. Clayton, having been a pupil of his and worked in association with him for a number of years, it is a privilege to be able to carry on, in some measure, the work that meant so much to him.

My thanks are due in this edition to Stanley Cox Medical Equipment of Rank Precision Industries Ltd and to Siemiens-Reigner-Werke AG of Germany, for information that they have supplied concerning microwave diathermy and other apparatus, to the Physiotherapy staff and students at King's College Hospital for their comments and advice, to Mrs J. Jefferies for reading the proofs, and to my publishers for their assistance in preparing this edition.

P. M. Scott

King's College Hospital,
London
June, 1969

CONTENTS

PART III

ACTINOTHERAPY AND OTHER RADIATIONS

PART I

ELECTROTHERAPY
DIRECT AND LOW FREQUENCY CURRENTS

I

STATIC ELECTRICITY

Structure of Matter

IN order to understand the principles of electricity some conception of the structure of matter is necessary.

ELEMENTS AND COMPOUNDS. Matter may be defined as "that which occupies space" and comprises a great number of different materials. These are built up from a comparatively small number of basic substances, the elements, which cannot be split into simpler materials. All other substances are compounds, which are formed by the union of two or more different elements. When this union takes place a completely new substance is formed, which may have quite different properties from its constituent elements. Common salt (sodium chloride) is a compound formed by the union of the elements sodium and chlorine and there is a great difference between its properties and those of the very active metal, sodium, and the suffocating gas, chlorine. When elements unite to form a compound a chemical change takes place and subsequently the elements cannot be separated by physical means.

An *element* may be defined as *a basic substance which cannot be split into simpler substances*. There are 92 natural elements and in addition a few which can be made artificially. A *compound* is a *substance formed by the union of two or more elements*. There is a vast number of compounds, ranging from the simple ones like sodium chloride to the very complex materials which form some organic substances.

MOLECULES AND ATOMS. A *molecule* is the *smallest particle of any substance, element or compound, that can exist alone*. If a grain of common salt were halved and the process repeated again and again, a minute particle would ultimately be reached which could not be further divided and still retain its properties.

3

This would be a molecule of sodium chloride, but as the material is a compound the molecule could be subdivided by chemical action into its constituent elements, sodium and chlorine. If a piece of an element were divided in a similar manner the smallest particle that could exist alone would be a molecule of that element. In the majority of cases this is the smallest particle of the element that can be obtained by any means, *i.e.* an atom, but there are a few elements, such as hydrogen, oxygen and chlorine, whose molecules can be divided on combination with other substances. The molecules of hydrogen and chlorine each consist of two atoms, but when they combine with each other two molecules of hydrochloric acid are formed, each consisting of one atom of hydrogen and one of chlorine. In this way the molecules of these elements are divided into smaller particles and an *atom* may be defined as *the smallest particle of an element that can take part in a chemical reaction.* Thus the atom and the molecule of the majority of elements are the same, but the molecules of a few elements consist of more than one atom. A molecule of a compound must contain a minimum of two atoms, as it cannot have less than two constituent elements and there must be at least one atom of each.

Structure of the Atom

PROTONS, NEUTRONS AND ELECTRONS. All atoms are built up from three basic types of particle; protons, neutrons and electrons. A proton is a particle with a very small mass, having a diameter of $1/2,000,000,000,000$ of an inch, and bearing a positive electric charge. A neutron has the same mass as a proton, but no electric charge, and an electron a still smaller mass, $1/1850$ that of a proton, and a negative electric charge.

ARRANGEMENT OF PARTICLES. The particles which form the atom are arranged like a minute solar system. The protons and neutrons are held together by a very strong cohesive force to form the central nucleus of the atom. This corresponds to the sun of the solar system and is very dense, containing practically all the mass of the atom within a very small space. The electrons revolve round the central nucleus at a very high speed, in orbits which resemble the pathways of the planets around the sun. They are held in the atom by the force of attraction exerted on them by the positively charged central nucleus, and the arrangement of the orbits follows a definite pattern, which is considered below. Fig. 1 shows the arrangement of the particles in a helium atom.

NUMBER OF PARTICLES. The number of protons in an atom is very important as it determines the element of which it is an atom. This is known as the atomic number of the element and for hydrogen is 1, helium 2, lithium 3, beryllium 4 and so on to uranium, the natural element which has the

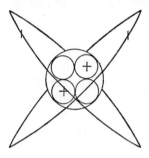

FIG. 1.—A HELIUM ATOM.

largest atom and an atomic number of 92. In the smaller atoms the number of neutrons is often equal to the number of protons, but the larger atoms usually contain more neutrons than protons. All atoms of a particular element do not necessarily contain the same number of neutrons. The nucleus of a hydrogen atom most often consists of one proton alone, but it may consist of one proton and one neutron, or of one proton and two neutrons. Atoms of an element which contain different numbers of neutrons are known as isotopes of that element. The protons and neutrons form practically all the mass of the atom and the number of these two particles together gives the atomic weight of the element.

The number of electrons in the atom normally equals the number of protons, so the positive and negative charges are equal and the atom is electrically neutral. Electrons can, however, be fairly easily displaced from or added to the atom.

If the atom gains electrons the number of electrons exceeds that of protons and the particle has a negative charge, while if electrons are lost the number of protons is greater than that of electrons and the charge is positive. Such charged particles are known as ions.

ARRANGEMENT OF ELECTRON ORBITS. The arrangement of the orbits in which the electrons circulate follows a definite plan. Several orbits may lie at the same distance from the central nucleus and these orbits form an electron "shell", as they constitute a "zone of negativeness" which it is difficult for other electrons to penetrate. The first shell, lying nearest to the central nucleus, contains up to two electrons, and must be completed before other shells are commenced. The single electron of the hydrogen atom is in this shell, which in all other atoms is complete. The second shell contains up to eight electrons and again is completed before a third shell is commenced. So the oxygen atom, with eight electrons, has two in the first shell and six in the second, while neon, with ten electrons, has two in the first shell and eight in the second, which is complete in this and all larger atoms. The plan is similar until there are eight electrons in the third shell, then becomes more complex, though still following a definite pattern. The arrangement of electron shells is shown diagrammatically in Fig. 2. The number in the centre of each atom is the atomic number while each of the surrounding circles represents an electron shell.

The arrangement of electron shells is important in determining the chemical properties of the elements. The atoms of the metals have one, two or three electrons in the outer shells, lithium, sodium and potassium, each with only one, having particularly similar properties. The halogens, fluorine, chlorine, bromine and iodine, all need one electron to complete the outer shell and the inert gases helium, neon, argon, krypton and xenon have a complete outer shell of electrons. The arrangement of the electron shells also plays a large part in the formation of ions and compounds, which is considered in Chapter 3, and is relevant to the principles of semiconductors (Chapter 7).

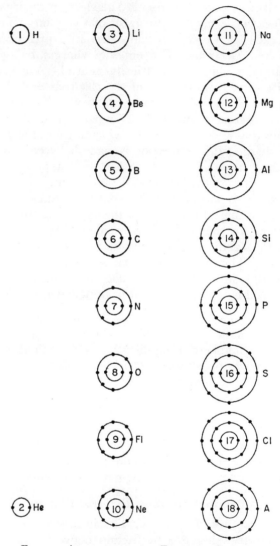

FIG. 2.—ARRANGEMENT OF ELECTRON SHELLS.

Theories of Electricity

THE ELECTRON THEORY. The electron theory is based on the fact that every object consists of a very large number of atoms, each of which normally has an equal number of protons and electrons. The opposite charges balance each other and the object is electrically neutral. A generator of electricity causes disturbance of the electrons and the object either gains electrons, becoming negatively charged, or loses electrons, becoming positively charged. In both cases the electricity is at rest on the object, which is said to have a static electric charge. If a connection is made between two objects, one with a negative and the other with a positive charge, electrons pass from the former to the latter until the charges are equalized. This flow of electrons constitutes an electric current which, according to the electron theory, passes from negative to positive. In the past it was usual to trace currents from positive to negative and the custom is still followed by some authorities. This is in accordance with the one fluid theory formulated below, but in this book the electron theory is followed and currents are traced from negative to positive.

THE ONE FLUID THEORY. This theory postulated that electricity was an invisible and weightless fluid, present on all objects but capable of being disturbed. If the fluid was at the normal level the object was electrically neutral, but an increase in the quantity of fluid gave rise to a positive charge, a decrease to a negative charge. If a connection was made between two oppositely charged objects fluid passed from the positively charged object to that with a negative charge, constituting an electric current. This theory has now been superseded by the electron theory but is worthy of consideration in that it explains the diversity of custom in tracing electric currents.

Production of an Electric Charge

CHARGING BY FRICTION. The simplest way of producing a static electric charge is by friction between two dissimilar materials. If a glass rod is rubbed with a piece of flannel it will subsequently attract small pieces of paper, the power of attraction for light objects being one of the properties of a charged body. To demonstrate charging by friction the materials chosen must be insulators. These do not readily allow electrons to move through them, so a charge produced on one part of the body is retained in that area. Conductors are materials which readily permit the movement of electrons and so any charge rapidly spreads throughout the object and its effects are less apparent. Similarly the materials must be dry, as water is a conductor of electricity and if the object is damp the charge leaks away.

When different materials are rubbed together electrons pass from one, which is left with a positive charge, to the other, which acquires a negative charge. The type of charge depends on the ease with which electrons can be displaced from the atoms of each material and those commonly used for these experiments can be arranged in order according to the charge that each will acquire. Of the following the material nearer the head of the list gains a positive charge:

Fur, flannel, glass, silk, sealing wax.

Thus a glass rod rubbed with flannel becomes negatively charged, the flannel being charged positively, but if the glass is rubbed with silk it becomes positively charged, the silk negatively.

OTHER METHODS OF PRODUCING ELECTRICITY. According to the law of conservation of energy, energy cannot be created or destroyed, though it can be converted from one form to another. Thus electricity must always be produced from some other form of energy. When it is produced by friction, mechanical energy is converted into electrical energy. Electricity can also be produced by chemical action, in cells; by electromagnetic induction, in a dynamo; from heat, in a thermocouple; and from radiant energy, in a photo-electric cell; but these methods are more commonly employed for the production of an electric current than a static charge.

Characteristics of a Charged Body

DISTRIBUTION OF THE CHARGE. The electric charge is always held on the surface of the object. The charged body may be regarded as striving continually to regain its neutral state, and it is from the surface that excess electrons can be lost. Similarly if the charge is positive it is the surface atoms that are deficient in electrons, as it is these atoms which can most easily gain more electrons. The charge tends to concentrate where the curvature of the surface is greatest. It spreads evenly over a sphere but concentrates at the edges and corners of a flat plate.

BEHAVIOUR OF LIKE AND UNLIKE CHARGES. Objects with like charges repel each other, those with unlike charges attract each other. If the hair is brushed vigorously on a dry day it crackles, an electric charge being produced by friction between the hair and the brush, and the individual hairs fly apart as they all have the same charge. A silk dress and a nylon petticoat tend to stick together, as friction between the two different materials gives them unlike electric charges.

TRANSMISSION OF ELECTRIC CHARGE. An electrically charged object can produce a charge on another object by contact or by induction. If two pith balls suspended on a silk thread are touched with a charged glass rod they fly apart and away from the rod (Fig. 3). If the rod has a negative charge

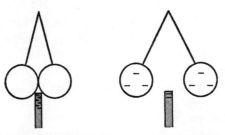

FIG. 3.—PITH BALLS TOUCHED WITH A
CHARGED ROD.

some of the excess electrons pass on to the pith balls, so that they also become negatively charged, and the like charges repel each other. When an object with a positive charge makes contact with one which is electrically neutral, some electrons pass from the uncharged to the charged body so that both are left with a deficiency. Thus a charge produced by contact is of the same nature as the original charge. It should be noted that it is always the electrons that move, the protons being firmly held within the central nuclei of the atoms.

ELECTROSTATIC INDUCTION. Induction may be defined as the production of electric or magnetic properties in one object by another without contact between them. So electrostatic induction is the production of a static electric charge in one object by another without contact between them. Other

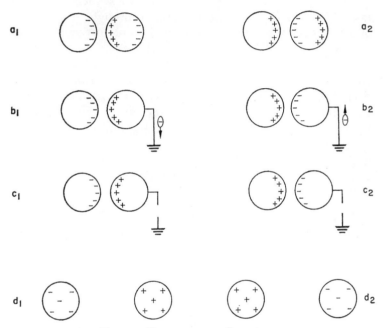

FIG. 4.—ELECTROSTATIC INDUCTION.

forms of induction are magnetic and electromagnetic induction, which are considered in subsequent chapters.

If a negatively charged object is brought close to, but not in contact with, one which is electrically neutral, electrons strive to pass from the former to the latter. They move to the side of the charged object adjacent to the neutral one and their influence causes a rearrangement of the electrons on the neutral object. These are repelled by the negative charge, leaving a positive charge on the side adjacent to the charged body and creating a negative one on the far side (Fig. $4a_1$). If the neutral object is now connected to earth the electrons are repelled to earth, which constitutes an inexhaustible reservoir of electrons, and the object is left with a positive charge (Fig. $4b_1$). The earth connection must now be broken, in order to prevent the return of the electrons (Fig. $4c_1$), and then when the originally uncharged object is removed from the influence of the charged one the charge spreads over its surface (Fig. $4d_1$). If the original charge is positive a similar sequence of events takes place. When the two objects are brought near to each other electrons on the neutral body are attracted by the positive charge. These create a negative charge on the surface of the body adjacent to the charged object, leaving a positive charge on the far side (Fig. $4a_2$). The neutral object is connected to earth, from which electrons are attracted to neutralise the positive charge on one side of the object (Fig. $4b_2$). The earth connection is then broken (Fig. $4c_2$) and when the object is removed from the influence of the original charged one the negative charge spreads over its surface (Fig. $4d_2$). Thus a charge produced by electrostatic induction is of the opposite nature to the one by which it is produced.

ATTRACTION FOR LIGHT OBJECTS. A charged object attracts an uncharged body which, if sufficiently light, moves towards it. This can be demonstrated with a charged glass rod and a scrap of paper, and is due to electrostatic induction. The charged object induces a charge of the opposite type on the adjacent surface of the uncharged one, the unlike charges attract each other and the objects move together.

ELECTRIC FIELD. The electric field is the area around a charged body in which the forces resulting from the charge are apparent. When one body is placed within the electric field of another the forces of attraction or repulsion are effective, and the closer the objects are together the more marked are these forces. Thus the electric field is most concentrated close to the charged object, becoming weaker as the distance from it increases.

The forces resulting from the charge act along definite lines, known as electric lines of force. These are the lines along which a free negative charge would move if placed within the electric field. They show certain characteristics:

They are considered to travel from negative to positive, this being the direction in which a free negative charge would move.

They tend to travel in straight lines, a straight line being the shortest distance between two points.

They behave as if they repel each other, as this would be the behaviour of two negative charges. This characteristic may be in opposition to the preceding one and the resulting distribution of the field is determined by a balance between the two tendencies.

They travel more easily through some materials than others, passing readily through conductors, less so through insulators.

As a result of these characteristics the lines of force around a charged sphere are straight lines radiating outwards and perpendicular to the surface (Fig. 5), while those around a less

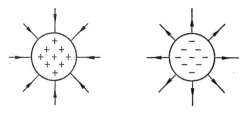

FIG. 5.—ELECTRIC FIELD AROUND A CHARGED SPHERE.

regular body are most concentrated at the edges or points where the charge is most concentrated (Fig. 6). Between two objects with opposite charges the lines of force pass from one to the other, but spread out somewhat, especially at the edges of the field, as they tend to repel each other (Fig. 7). If a conductor, such as a metal sphere, is placed within the field, the lines of force concentrate on it because they can pass through it easily (Fig. 8).

The behaviour of electric lines of force is of considerable importance to the physiotherapist as they are utilised when applying short-wave diathermy by the condenser field method.

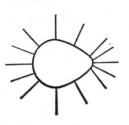

FIG. 6.—ELECTRIC FIELD AROUND AN IRREGULAR BODY.

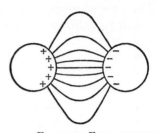

FIG. 7.—ELECTRIC FIELD BETWEEN OPPOSITELY CHARGED OBJECTS.

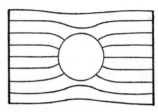

FIG. 8.—ELECTRIC LINES OF FORCE BETWEEN TWO CHARGED METAL PLATES WITH A CONDUCTOR IN THE FIELD.

Potential and Capacity

ELECTRICAL POTENTIAL. The properties exhibited by a charged body result from the stored up, or potential, energy of its electric charge, and its electrical condition is referred to as its electrical potential. An object with excess electrons is said to be at a negative potential, one with a deficiency at a positive potential. The earth is so large that it can receive or give up electrons indefinitely yet never show the properties of a charged body, so it is said to be at zero potential and is taken as the standard from which potential is measured. If an object with excess electrons is connected to earth the extra electrons pass from it to earth, while if one with a deficiency is connected to earth it will attract electrons from earth until it also is electrically neutral. Thus an object with a negative potential is one which tends to give up electrons to earth, while one with a positive potential is one which tends to receive electrons from earth.

FACTORS DETERMINING POTENTIAL. The unit of potential is the volt, which is defined in Chapter 2. The greater the electrical potential of an object the more marked are the properties resulting from the charge. When considering the magnitude of potential it is often convenient to think of it in terms of one of these properties, *i.e.* the greater the potential the greater is the repelling power for a like charge. The magnitude of the potential depends on:

1. The quantity of electricity with which the object is charged.

2. The capacity of the object.

Quantity of electricity is measured in coulombs, one coulomb being a definite number of electrons. If two identical objects are charged with different quantities of electricity the one with the greater quantity of electricity has more stored-up energy than the other. This gives it a greater repelling power for a like charge and so it has the greater potential of the two. In Fig. 9 A is charged with more electricity than B, so has a greater potential. Thus the potential varies directly with the quantity of electricity with which the object is charged.

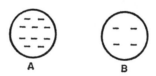

FIG. 9.—OBJECTS CHARGED WITH DIFFERENT QUANTITIES OF ELECTRICITY.

The capacity of an object is its ability to hold an electric charge and depends on:

1. The material. Some materials hold electricity more readily than others, conductors having the greatest power of storing a charge, and an object of such a material tends to have a large capacity.

2. The surface area. The charge is always on the surface of

the object so the greater the surface area the greater is the capacity.

If two objects of different capacities are charged with the same quantity of electricity, the charge is more concentrated on the smaller than on the larger. The pressure developed by the electricity on the smaller is therefore greater than that on the larger, and this gives it a greater repelling power for a like charge, and so a greater potential, than the object with the larger capacity. Fig. 10 shows two such objects. B has a smaller capacity than A and is charged to a greater potential by the same quantity of electricity. Thus the potential varies inversely with the capacity of the object. In order to charge two objects of different capacities to the same potential, the larger must receive a greater quantity of electricity than the smaller (Fig. 11).

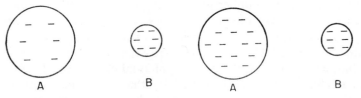

FIG. 10.—OBJECTS OF DIFFERENT CAPACITIES CHARGED WITH EQUAL QUANTITIES OF ELECTRICITY.

FIG. 11.—OBJECTS OF DIFFERENT CAPACITIES CHARGED TO THE SAME POTENTIAL.

Thus the *electrical potential varies directly with the quantity of the charge and inversely with the capacity of the object*. This is expressed by the formula:

$$E = \frac{Q}{C}$$ where E = potential measured in volts.

Q = quantity of charge measured in coulombs.

C = capacity measured in farads.

MEASUREMENT OF CAPACITY. The capacity of a jug can be measured by the quantity of a liquid that it will hold, but this method is not suitable for electricity. Provided that there is sufficient power available it is possible to force an indefinite quantity of electricity on to an object. The effect of increasing the quantity of electricity is to increase the pressure of the charge and so the electrical potential of the object. This may be compared to pumping up a tyre. Provided that sufficient force is available more and more air can be pumped into the tyre, the effect being to increase the pressure. The smaller the capacity of an object, the more rapidly is the pressure built up and the greater is the potential produced by a given quantity of electricity. Similarly a certain quantity of air produces a greater pressure in a bicycle tyre than in a motor tyre. Thus the potential produced by a given quantity of electricity varies inversely with the capacity of the object, and the capacity can be assessed by the potential produced by a definite quantity of electricity.

The unit of capacity is the *farad*, which is *the capacity of an object which is charged to a potential of one volt by one coulomb of electricity*. This unit is very large and the microfarad, which is one millionth of a farad, is more commonly used.

DIFFERENCE OF POTENTIAL. When two objects are in a different state of electric charge a difference of potential is said to exist between them. To achieve this one may have a negative and the other a positive potential, one may be charged negatively or positively and the other be at zero potential, or both may have a charge of the same nature but one be charged to a greater potential than the other. If objects between which there is a difference of potential are connected by a conductor electrons pass from the more negative to the less negative until the objects are at the same potential. The movement of electrons constitutes an electric current and is produced by a force, known as an electromotive force (EMF), which results from a difference of potential. The EMF cannot, however, produce a current unless there is a pathway, or circuit, through which the electrons are able to move. So the two essentials for the production of an electric current are a circuit and a difference of potential between the ends of that circuit.

CURRENT ELECTRICITY

The Electric Current

AN electric current is a flow of electrons and is produced when a difference of potential exists between the ends of a conducting pathway. The essentials for the production of an electric current are:

1. A difference of potential (P.D.).
2. A pathway along which electrons can move.

ELECTROMOTIVE FORCE. A difference of potential gives rise to a force, known as an electromotive force (EMF), which tends to produce a movement of electrons. If a pathway is provided the EMF produces a flow of electrons, but if there is no pathway, so that no current can pass, the force still exists. The greater the P.D. the greater is the EMF, and both are measured in the same unit, the volt. A *volt is that EMF which when applied to a conductor with a resistance of one ohm produces a current of one ampere.* The other units involved in this definition are explained below.

Electrons move only so long as a P.D. exists between the ends of the pathway, *i.e.* so long as the EMF is maintained. A P.D. can be produced by friction, but when a pathway is completed the charges quickly neutralise each other and current ceases to flow. Other methods of producing a P.D., and so an EMF, are by chemical action, in cells; by electromagnetic induction, in a dynamo; by heat, in a thermocouple; and from radiant energy, in a photo-electric cell. With all these methods the P.D. is maintained in spite of the electron flow. As fast as electrons move away from the negative end of the conductor they are replaced by others from the generator, while those which reach the positive end are drawn away by the generator. Thus the P.D. is maintained and current continues to flow.

RESISTANCE. A pathway through which electrons can move is known as a circuit, and the conductor of which it is made offers some impedance to the movement of electrons. The amount of this resistance depends on:

1. *The material of the conductor.* Some materials allow electrons to move through them more easily than others, and so have a low resistance. A characteristic of the atoms of the metals is that some of the electrons rotate in orbits at a considerable distance from the central nuclei, and so are not strongly held by them. These electrons may come under the influence of the nuclei of adjacent atoms so that, though the metal as a whole contains an equal number of protons and electrons, some electrons are drifting freely without being connected to a definite atom. When a P.D. is applied the free electrons move away from the more negative and towards the more positive end of the conductor, constituting an electric current. The less strongly the electrons are held by the central nuclei, the greater the number that are drifting freely and are available to move, so the lower is the resistance of the material. This type of current, which occurs in metals and carbon, is called a conduction current. In other materials the electron movement takes place in a different manner and may constitute a convection current or a displacement current. These types of current are considered later.

2. *The length of the pathway.* If electrons have to move through a long pathway they encounter more impedance than in a short one, so resistance varies directly with the length of the conductor.

3. *Cross-sectional area of the conductor.* The greater the cross-sectional area of the pathway, the more room there is for the electrons to move, so the resistance varies inversely with the cross-sectional area.

4. *Temperature.* In most materials rise in temperature increases the resistance of the conductor. Molecules are always in a state of vibration and this movement, which tends to impede the flow of electrons, is increased by heat. An exception to this effect on resistance occurs in certain semiconductors (Chapter 7).

The impedance to the electron flow which is determined by

the material, physical dimensions and temperature of the conductor is termed the ohmic resistance. Provided that the temperature does not vary the ohmic resistance is a constant factor for any particular conductor. The unit of resistance is the *ohm* which is *the resistance offered by a column of mercury* 106·3 *centimetres long and one square millimetre in cross-sectional area at* 0° *C.* or *the resistance offered by* 50 *yards of copper wire one square millimetre in cross-sectional area at N.T.P.*

In addition to the ohmic resistance the flow of current in a circuit is impeded by inductive reactance (Chapter 5) and capacitive reactance (Chapter 6).

INTENSITY OF CURRENT. The rate of flow of electrons through a conductor is known as the intensity of the current. The rate of flow of water can be measured in pints per minute, *i.e.* quantity per unit time, and the rate of flow of electrons is measured in a similar manner. The unit of quantity of electricity is the coulomb and the rate of flow of electrons, or intensity of current, is measured in coulombs per second. The *ampere* is the unit of intensity of current and is *a rate of flow of electrons of one coulomb per second*. An alternative definition of the ampere is *that intensity of current which when passed through a solution of silver nitrate in water deposits* 0·001118 *gramme of silver per second at the cathode*. A milliampere is one thousandth of an ampere and is a unit often used in medical work. A coulomb is a definite number of electrons and the definition of the coulomb can be based on that of the ampere. A *coulomb* is *the number of electrons that pass if a current of one ampere flows for one second*.

The intensity of an electric current depends on:

1. The electromotive force. The greater the force applied the greater is the rate of flow of electrons, so the intensity of the current varies directly with the EMF, that is with the P.D. between the ends of the conductor.

2. The resistance. The greater the impedance offered to the electron movement, the less is the rate of flow of electrons. So the intensity of the current varies inversely with the resistance of the conductor.

This may be compared with the flow of water, the rate of flow depending on the force which is causing it to move and on the resistance offered by the channel through which it is passing.

OHM'S LAW. The relationship between EMF, resistance and intensity of current is stated in Ohm's law, but may be more simply expressed as:

The intensity of an electric current varies directly with the EMF and inversely with the resistance of the conductor.

Ohm's law is expressed by the formula:

$I = \frac{E}{R}$ where I = intensity of current measured in amperes.
E = EMF measured in volts.
R = resistance measured in ohms.

The formula can also be written:

$$E = IR \quad \text{or} \quad R = \frac{E}{I}$$

Thus if two of the factors are known, the third can be calculated. As there is a definite relationship between the EMF, resistance and intensity of current, and the units of resistance and intensity of current have been defined, the definition of the volt can be based on the other two factors.

DIRECT AND ALTERNATING CURRENTS. A generator of electricity may keep one end of the circuit negatively charged and the other positive. Then the electrons always move in the same direction and a direct current (D.C.) is produced. Another type of generator, namely the alternating current dynamo, causes a continual change in the polarity of the ends of the circuit. At first one end is negative and the other

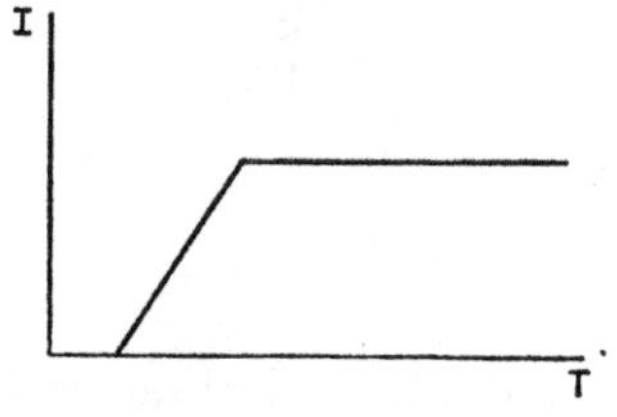

FIG. 12.—DIRECT CURRENT.

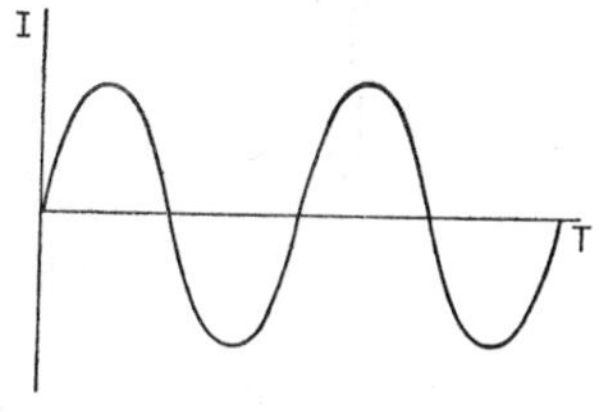

FIG. 13.—ALTERNATING CURRENT.

positive, then the polarity is reversed. The electrons move first in one direction and then in the other, constituting an alternating current (A.C.). Each to and fro movement of electrons is one cycle and the frequency of the current is the number of cycles per unit time. This varies under different circumstances but the frequency of the A.C. obtained from the main supply is usually 50 cycles per second. Figs. 12 and 13 show the graphs representing direct and alternating currents.

Resistances in Series and Parallel

Component parts forming a circuit may be connected together in two different ways, in series or in parallel with each other.

RESISTANCES IN SERIES (Fig. 14). The resistances are connected together end to end so that the current has only one pathway. Consequently the current is compelled to pass through each of the resistances in turn and the *total resistance is the sum of the individual resistances*.

This is expressed by the formula:

$$R = r_1 + r_2 + r_3 \ldots r_n$$

where R is the total resistance, r_1, r_2, r_3 etc. the individual resistances and n the number of resistances.

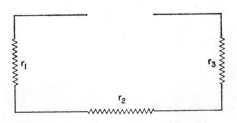

FIG. 14.—RESISTANCES IN SERIES.

As all the current has to pass through all the resistances *the intensity of current is the same throughout the circuit*. A greater force is necessary to produce this current in the parts of the circuit with a high resistance than in those with a low resistance. Consequently the force, or potential, drops by a greater amount across the high resistances than across the low ones. So *the potential drop across each resistance is directly proportional to its resistance.*

The addition of more resistances in series increases the total resistance and reduces the intensity of current in all parts of the circuit.

The following example illustrates these points:

Three resistances are wired in series with each other

$$r_1 = 75 \text{ ohms.} \quad r_2 = 5 \text{ ohms.} \quad r_3 = 20 \text{ ohms.}$$
$$R = r_1 + r_2 + r_3 = 75 + 5 + 20 = 100 \text{ ohms.}$$

Suppose an EMF of 200 volts is applied

$$\text{By Ohm's law } I = \frac{E}{R} = \frac{200}{100} = 2 \text{ amps.}$$

This intensity of current is the same in all the resistances.

Thus the P.D. across each:

r_1. $E = IR = 2 \times 75 = 150$ v.

r_2. $E = IR = 2 \times 5 = 10$ v.

r_3. $E = IR = 2 \times 20 = 40$ v.

In the above example r_1 constitutes three-quarters of the total resistance and the P.D. across it is three-quarters of the total voltage. Similarly r_2 forms one-twentieth of the total resistance, and the P.D. across it is one-twentieth of the voltage, while r_3 forms one-fifth of the resistance and the P.D. across it is one-fifth of the total voltage.

If a fourth resistance, r_4, of 100 ohms were added in series with these three resistances, then the total resistance would be increased:

$$75 + 5 + 20 + 100 = 200 \text{ ohms.}$$

This would cause a decrease in the intensity of current in all parts of the circuit:

$$I = \frac{E}{R} = \frac{200}{200} = 1 \text{ ampere.}$$

and an alteration in the P.D. across each resistance:

r_1. $E = IR = 1 \times 75 = 75$ v.
r_2. $E = IR = 1 \times 5 = 5$ v.
r_3. $E = IR = 1 \times 20 = 20$ v.
r_4. $E = IR = 1 \times 100 = 100$ v.

The P.D. across r_3 is now one-tenth instead of one-fifth of the whole, as r_3 now constitutes only one-tenth of the total resistance, and there are similar alterations in the P.D. across the other resistances. Thus the P.D. across each resistance is determined not by its actual resistance but by the proportion that it forms of the total resistance of the circuit.

RESISTANCES IN PARALLEL (OR SHUNT) (Fig. 15). The resistances are connected so that they tap the main circuit at two points, and thus provide alternative pathways for the current. As the pathways are taken from the same two points on the circuit, the *potential drop across all of them is the same*. The intensity of current in each part varies directly with the P.D.

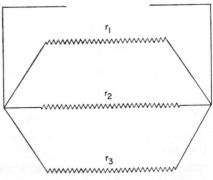

FIG. 15.—RESISTANCES IN PARALLEL.

and inversely with the resistance of the part of the pathway. As the P.D. across all is the same *the intensity of current in each of the parallel pathways is inversely proportional to the resistance of the pathway*. Thus the intensity of current is greatest in the low resistance pathways, least in those of high resistance. The intensity of current in each pathway is unaffected by that in the others, and the total intensity of current is the sum of the intensities in the parallel pathways.

The connection of resistances in parallel has the same effect as increasing the cross-sectional area of the conductor. This reduces the *total resistance*, which is *less than that of any of the individual resistances*. To calculate the total resistance the following points should be considered:

The total intensity of current is equal to the sum of the intensities in the different parts,

$$\text{i.e. } I = i_1 + i_2 + i_3 \ldots i_n$$

where I is the total intensity of current, i_1, i_2, i_3, etc. the intensities in the different parts.

$$\text{By Ohm's law } I = \frac{E}{R}$$

$$\text{so } \frac{E}{R} = \frac{E}{r_1} + \frac{E}{r_2} + \frac{E}{r_3} \ldots \frac{E}{r_n}$$

Dividing through by E

$$\frac{I}{R} = \frac{I}{r_1} + \frac{I}{r_2} + \frac{I}{r_3} \ldots \frac{I}{r_n}$$

This formula is used to calculate the total resistance of the circuit.

The addition of further parallel pathways serves to reduce the resistance of the circuit as a whole, and increases the total intensity of current.

The following example illustrates these points:

Three resistances are wired in parallel with each other

$$r_1 = 5 \text{ ohms. } r_2 = 10 \text{ ohms. } r_3 = 20 \text{ ohms.}$$

To calculate the total resistance:

$$\frac{I}{R} = \frac{I}{5} + \frac{I}{10} + \frac{I}{20} = \frac{7}{20}$$

$$\text{so } R = 2\tfrac{6}{7} \text{ ohms.}$$

Thus the total resistance is less than any of the individual resistances.

Suppose an EMF of 20 volts is applied

$$\text{By Ohm's law } I = \frac{E}{R} = \frac{20}{2\frac{6}{7}} = 7 \text{ amps.}$$

There is a P.D. of 20 v. across each pathway, so the intensity of the current in each can be calculated:

$$r_1 = 5 \text{ ohms. } i_1 = \frac{20}{5} = 4 \text{ amps.}$$

$$r_2 = 10 \text{ ohms. } i_2 = \frac{20}{10} = 2 \text{ amps.}$$

$$r_3 = 20 \text{ ohms. } i_3 = \frac{20}{20} = 1 \text{ amp.}$$

and $I = 4 + 2 + 1 = 7$ amps.

Thus the total intensity of current is equal to the sum of the intensities in the different parts, while the intensity of current in each of the parallel pathways varies inversely with its resistance.

If an additional pathway, r_4, with a resistance of 2 ohms were added in parallel to the above pathways, this would reduce the total resistance of the circuit:

$$\frac{1}{R} = \frac{1}{5} + \frac{1}{10} + \frac{1}{20} + \frac{1}{2} = \frac{17}{20}$$

so $R = 1\frac{3}{17}$ ohms.

Consequently the total intensity of current in the circuit would be increased:

$$I = \frac{E}{R} = \frac{20}{1\frac{3}{17}} = 17 \text{ amps.}$$

The P.D. across, and the resistance of, the other pathways is not affected so the intensity of current in each of them remains the same as before, and the total intensity of current is increased by that obtained in r_4.

$$i_4 = \frac{E}{r_4} = \frac{20}{2} = 10 \text{ amps.}$$

and $I = 4 + 2 + 1 + 10 = 17$ amps.

Devices for Regulating Intensity of Current

The intensity of an electric current varies directly with the EMF and inversely with the resistance of the pathway. Thus the intensity of current in a circuit can be varied by altering either the EMF or the resistance. These methods are employed in the potential divider, also known as a potentiometer or shunt rheostat, and the variable resistance or series rheostat. The construction of these two devices is the same. The difference between them lies in the method of wiring into the circuit.

CONSTRUCTION OF THE RHEOSTAT. The rheostat consists of a coil of wire of some material offering a fairly high resistance, such as german silver, wound on a block of insulating material. This may be straight or circular in shape. The coil is varnished to insulate the turns of wire from each other, but the varnish is scraped off where a moving contact touches the wire. With the straight type this contact slides along a metal bar lying beside the coil, while with the circular one it is attached to a revolving knob pivoted in the centre of the coil.

THE VARIABLE RESISTANCE. As in Fig. 16, wires from one end of the resistance coil and from the moving contact are connected respectively to the source of supply and to the circuit in which the current is to be regulated. Thus this circuit is in series with the coil. When the contact is at the right hand end of the coil (W in Fig. 16) the whole of the resistance is included in the circuit. Resistance is maximal and intensity of current minimal. As the contact is moved to the left, part of the coil is cut out of the circuit, the resistance is reduced, and the intensity of current increases. When the contact reaches the left hand end of the coil (S) the resistance is at a minimum and the intensity of current maximal. While suitable for regulating current supplied to certain pieces of apparatus, such as U.V.R. lamps, this device cannot be used for regulating the current to a patient. The resistance of the circuit is never so great that the intensity of current is reduced to zero, so as soon as the apparatus is turned on current flows, and a patient in the circuit would receive a shock.

THE POTENTIAL DIVIDER. As in Fig. 17, the two ends of

the coil are connected to the source of supply. The circuit in which the current is to be regulated is taken in parallel to this coil, by one wire from one end of the coil, marked "weak" (W in Fig. 17), and one wire from the sliding contact. When the current is flowing from the supply there is an even potential drop along the resistance coil. If, for example, an EMF of 60

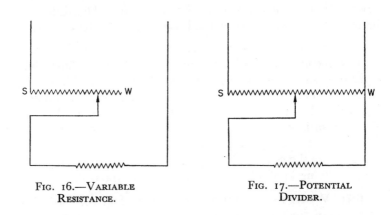

Fig. 16.—Variable Resistance.

Fig. 17.—Potential Divider.

volts is applied to a coil containing 60 turns of wire, there is a P.D. of 1 volt across each turn of wire. When the moving contact is at the end of the coil marked W, the two wires to the parallel circuit are in contact with the same point of the main circuit, so there is no P.D. between them and no current flows in the parallel circuit. As the contact is moved away from W the two ends of the parallel circuit are connected to different points on the coil, so a P.D. exists between them and current flows in the parallel circuit. In the above example, when there is one turn of wire between the contact and the point W, there is a P.D. of 1 volt between these two points and so across the parallel circuit, when two turns of wire, 2 volts, etc. Thus as the contact moves along the coil towards the end marked "strong" (S in Fig. 17) the P.D. between the ends of the parallel circuit increases and so does the current in this circuit. When the contact reaches S the P.D. across the parallel circuit is the same as that across the coil and the intensity of current in the parallel circuit is at its maximum. This device enables the current to be regulated from zero, so is suitable for controlling the current supplied to a patient.

Electrical Energy and Power

Any system which is capable of doing work is said to possess energy, which can therefore be defined as ability to do work. There are various forms of energy: heat, sound, magnetism, electricity and radiant, mechanical, nuclear and chemical energy, and although energy cannot be created or destroyed, it can be converted from one form to another. Thus electrical energy is always obtained from some other form of energy and can in its turn produce other types of energy; it is converted into mechanical energy in an electric motor and into heat in electric radiators, cookers and irons.

When energy is converted from one form to another work is done. The definition of work is usually related to mechanical energy, and work is said to be done whenever a force moves its point of application. So work is done when an electromotive force causes a movement of electrons, *i.e.* whenever an electric current flows. The amount of work done by any system depends on the magnitude of the force and the amount of movement that it produces, being determined by the product of these two factors. So the amount of work done by an electric current depends on the product of the EMF and the quantity of electrons moved. When an EMF of 1 volt moves 1 coulomb of electrons, the work done is 1 joule, *i.e.*

$$\text{work done} = E \times Q \text{ joules,}$$
where E = EMF measured in volts.
 Q = Quantity of electrons measured in coulombs.

The power of a system is its rate of doing work, so the power of an electric current depends on the work that it does in a given time. If an EMF of 1 volt moves 1 coulomb of electrons, the work done is 1 joule, and if this work is done in 1 second the power is 1 watt. So *1 watt* is the rate of doing work, or *power of 1 joule per second.* In this case the rate of movement of electrons is 1 coulomb per second, so the intensity of current is 1 ampere, and a watt may be defined as the *power of a current of 1 ampere at an EMF of 1 volt.* If the EMF is increased to 2 volts, the power is doubled, *i.e.* 2 watts. Increasing the intensity of current has the same effect, so a current of 2 amperes with a force of 2 volts represents a power of 4 watts. Thus power is calculated by multiplying the EMF, in volts, by the intensity of current, in amperes, *i.e.*

$$\text{watts} = \text{volts} \times \text{amperes}.$$

This may be likened to a stream of water coming from a hose pipe. The ability of the water to displace any object in its path, *i.e.* to do work, depends on both the pressure, or force of the water and on the quantity of water emitted in a given time, *i.e.* the rate of flow. A large volume at a high pressure is more effective than either a small stream at a high pressure or a large volume at a low pressure.

The efficiency of electrical equipment depends on its rate of doing work, *i.e.* its power, so is indicated by the wattage. A 100 watt electric light bulb gives more light than a 40 watt bulb. This subject is considered further in Chapter 8.

The amount of work done by any system is determined by:

(1) the rate of doing work, *i.e.* the power, and
(2) the time for which the work is done.

E.g. if a man is sawing logs at the rate of 50 logs per hour, the total number of logs sawn depends on the time for which the activity is maintained, *i.e.* 1 hour, 50 logs, 2 hours, 100 logs etc.

The quantity of work done is proportional to the amount of energy expended, so quantity of electrical energy can be calculated by considering the electric power and the time for which it is used.

$$\text{Energy} = \text{power} \times \text{time}.$$

The Board of Trade unit of electrical energy is the *Kilowatt Hour,* which is the amount of energy needed to maintain an output of 1,000 watts for 1 hour. The same amount of energy would be required to provide 500 watts for 2 hours, 2,000 watts for half an hour etc.

Thermal Effect of an Electric Current

When electrical energy is converted into some other form of energy, physical effects are produced. These include the thermal, chemical (Chapter 3), and magnetic (Chapter 4) effects.

When a current is passed through a conductor part of the electrical energy is converted into heat, and *Joule's law* states that *the amount of heat produced in a conductor is proportional to the square of the intensity of current, the resistance and the time for which the current flows.*

As the electrical energy is converted into heat, work is done and the amount of heat produced depends on the amount of work done. This depends on the power, or rate of doing work and on the time for which the power is exercised. Thus:

$$\text{work done} = \text{watts} \times \text{time}$$
$$= E \times I \times t \text{ joules,}$$

where E = EMF measured in volts.
   I = Intensity of current measured in amperes.
   t = Time measured in seconds.

By Ohm's law, E = I.R.

So work done = $I \times R \times I \times t$.
   = I^2Rt joules.

One calorie of heat is produced by 4·2 joules of work.

$$\text{So heat generated} = \frac{I^2Rt}{4\cdot2}\text{calories.}$$

Joule's law can be applied to ascertain the heat produced in different parts of a circuit. When resistances are wired in series with each other the intensity of current and the time for which it flows are the same for all parts of the circuit. Therefore the amount of heat generated in each part depends on the resistance, with which it varies directly. So more heat is produced in a high resistance than in a low one.

E.g. two resistances wired in series with each other.

$$r_1 = 10 \text{ ohms.} \quad r_2 = 20 \text{ ohms.}$$

An EMF of 90 volts is applied.

Total resistance $= 10+20 = 30$ ohms.

Intensity of current throughout the circuit:

$$I = \frac{E}{R} = \frac{90}{30} = 3 \text{ amperes.}$$

Heat produced in $r_1 = \dfrac{i_1^2 \times r_1 \times t}{4 \cdot 2}$

$$= \frac{3 \times 3 \times 10 \times t}{4 \cdot 2} = \frac{90t}{4 \cdot 2} \text{ calories}$$

Heat produced in $r_2 = \dfrac{i_2^2 \times r_2 \times t}{4 \cdot 2}$

$$= \frac{3 \times 3 \times 20 \times t}{4 \cdot 2} = \frac{180t}{4 \cdot 2} \text{ calories}$$

Thus more heat is generated in r_2 than in r_1.

When resistances are wired in parallel with each other the intensity of current in each is inversely proportional to the resistance. The time is the same for all parts of the circuit, but where the resistance is high the intensity of current is low and vice versa. The heat produced is proportional to the resistance, but to the square of the intensity of current. Therefore the intensity of current has more effect on the heat production than has the resistance, and more heat is generated in a low than in a high resistance.

E.g. two resistances are wired in parallel with each other.

$$r_1 = 10 \text{ ohms.} \quad r_2 = 20 \text{ ohms.}$$

An EMF of 100 volts is applied.

The intensity of current in each:

$$i_1 = \frac{E}{r_2} = \frac{100}{10} = 10 \text{ amps.}$$

$$i_2 = \frac{E}{r_2} = \frac{100}{20} = 5 \text{ amps.}$$

Heat produced in $r_1 = \dfrac{i_1^2 \times r_1 \times t}{4 \cdot 2}$

$$= \frac{10 \times 10 \times 10 \times t}{4 \cdot 2} = \frac{1000t}{4 \cdot 2} \text{ calories}$$

Heat produced in $r_2 = \dfrac{i_2^2 \times r_2 \times t}{4 \cdot 2}$

$$= \frac{5 \times 5 \times 20 \times t}{4 \cdot 2} = \frac{500t}{4 \cdot 2} \text{ calories}$$

Thus more heat is generated in r_1 than in r_2.

C

3

CHEMICAL EFFECTS OF CURRENT

Ions and Compounds

FORMATION OF IONS. An *ion* is *an atom or group of atoms bearing a negative or positive electric charge.* Atoms normally contain an equal number of protons and electrons and so are electrically neutral. The protons, together with the neutrons, form the central nucleus, and the electrons revolve round this in orbits, the orbits being arranged in definite electron "shells" (Chapter 1). In every atom there are two tendencies, one for the number of electrons to equal that of protons, the other for the outer electron shell to be a complete one, but only in the case of the inert gases is the number of

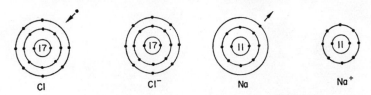

| FIG. 18.—FORMATION OF A CHLORINE ION. $Cl + e = Cl^-$. | FIG. 19.—FORMATION OF A SODIUM ION. $Na - e = Na^+$. |

electrons such that these two tendencies can be fulfilled at the same time. Atoms of other elements can acquire a complete outer electron shell only by gaining or losing electrons. In this case the number of electrons no longer equals that of protons and the particle becomes electrically charged, forming an ion. If the outer electron shell is more than half complete, but still lacking some electrons, the atom tends to gain electrons. When this occurs it has more negative than positive charges and forms a negative ion. A chlorine atom has 7 electrons in its third shell, so readily acquires one more electron to form an ion bearing a single negative charge (Fig. 18). If the outer shell is less than half complete the atom tends to lose the electrons from this shell, so that its outermost electron shell is a complete one. It then has an excess of positive over negative charges and forms a positive ion. A sodium atom has one electron in its outer shell and readily loses this to form an ion with a single positive charge (Fig. 19). It may be necessary for the atom to

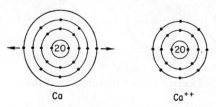

Ca   Ca^{++}

FIG. 20.—FORMATION OF A CALCIUM ION.
$Ca - 2e = Ca^{++}$.

gain or lose more than one electron for the outer shell to be a complete one. A calcium atom has two electrons in its outermost shell, so tends to lose both of these to form an ion with a double positive charge (Fig. 20). The atoms of hydrogen and the metals tend to lose electrons, so forming positive ions, while the acid and hydroxyl radicals (page 37) gain electrons and form negative ions.

FORMATION OF COMPOUNDS. A compound is a substance formed by the union of two or more elements. There are two ways in which this union may take place:

Electrovalent compounds are compounds whose molecules consist of the ions of the constituent elements held together by the attraction of their opposite electrical charges. When an atom of sodium, which tends to lose one electron, comes in contact with an atom of chlorine, which requires one electron to form a complete outer electron shell, an electron passes from the sodium to the chlorine. Two oppositely charged ions are formed, which are subsequently held together by the attraction of their opposite charges. Thus a molecule of sodium chloride (NaCl) consists of one sodium ion, bearing a single positive charge, and one chlorine ion, with a single negative charge (Fig. 21). A calcium atom has two electrons available and if it comes in contact with chlorine it gives up those electrons to chlorine atoms. Each chlorine atom needs only one electron, so one is given to each of two chlorine atoms. Two chlorine ions, each with a single negative charge, and one calcium ion, with a double positive charge, are formed. The ions are held together

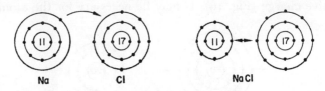

Na   Cl   NaCl

FIG. 21.—FORMATION OF A MOLECULE OF SODIUM CHLORIDE.

by the attraction of their opposite charges and constitute a molecule of calcium chloride ($CaCl_2$).

Substances formed in this way are the strong acids, *e.g.* sulphuric, hydrochloric and nitric acid, the strong alkalis, *e.g.* potassium and sodium hydroxide, and all true salts.

Covalent compounds are compounds whose molecules consist of atoms of the constituent elements held together by shared electron bonds. The atoms join together and "share" electrons so that each of them has a complete outer electron shell. The manner in which this occurs is not fully understood, but the sharing of the electrons forms a bond which unites the particles. A molecule of water, consisting of one atom of oxygen and two of hydrogen, is formed in this manner. The oxygen atom requires two electrons to complete its outer shell, each hydrogen atom one. The oxygen atom shares one electron with each hydrogen atom, so completing their outer shells, and receives in exchange a share in the electrons of the hydrogen atoms. Thus it also has a complete outer electron shell (Fig. 22).

Compounds formed in this way are the weak acids, *e.g.* carbonic acid, the weak alkalis, *e.g.* zinc hydroxide, the metallic oxides and organic compounds.

Other particles may consist of atoms united, like those of the covalent compounds, by shared electron bonds. The molecules of elements which contain more than one atom are formed in this way, those of hydrogen and oxygen being examples, and the particles known as radicals consist of atoms united in the same manner.

Radicals are groups of atoms which are frequently found in union with each other. Examples are the carbonate (CO_3), sulphate (SO_4) and hydroxyl (OH) radicals. The atoms of the group are united by shared electron bonds but do not achieve a complete outer electron shell. Thus they tend to acquire more electrons and form negative ions. They behave like the atoms of elements and can enter into the formation of electrovalent

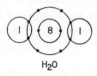

H₂O

FIG. 22.—A WATER
MOLECULE.

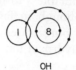

OH

FIG. 23.—A HYDROXYL
RADICAL.

or of covalent compounds. The hydroxyl radical (Fig. 23) consists of one atom of oxygen and one of hydrogen each sharing one electron with the other atom but still lacking one electron in the outer shell. This radical tends to acquire one electron and so form an ion with a single negative charge. It can enter into the formation of electrovalent compounds, *e.g.* sodium hydroxide (NaOH) and covalent compounds, *e.g.* zinc hydroxide $(Zn(OH)_2)$.

DISSOCIATION OF MOLECULES. The molecules of the electrovalent compounds each consist of two or more separate ions which are held together by the attraction of their opposite electrical charges. These molecules are said to be in a state of dissociation, which becomes more apparent when the substance is dissolved in water. When this occurs the molecules are less tightly packed together than when the substance is in solid form, and the ions drift away from each other.

The particles forming the molecules of the covalent compounds are normally united by shared electron bonds, but some of the molecules of some of the covalent compounds may split up into ions and assume a structure resembling that of the molecules of the electrovalent compounds. That is, there may be some dissociation of molecules. This occurs in the weak acids and alkalis, in water, and in some organic compounds, but not in other covalent compounds.

In water each molecule that dissociates forms one hydrogen and one hydroxyl ion:

$$H_2O \rightleftharpoons H^+ + OH^-$$

Each hydrogen ion so formed unites with a water molecule to form a hydronium ion (H_3O^+), but this does not affect the basic principle and it is most convenient to consider hydrogen ions, although in fact each is attached to a water molecule. Thus in pure water the number of hydrogen ions is equal to that of hydroxyl ions, *i.e.*:

Hydrogen ion concentration = hydroxyl ion concentration.

The number of water molecules which dissociate is very small, so there are few ions relative to undissociated water molecules.

ACID AND ALKALINE REACTIONS. Hydrogen ions are responsible for the properties of an acid, hydroxyl ions for those of an alkali. In pure water there are the same number of hydrogen and hydroxyl ions, so their properties counteract each other and the reaction is neutral. An acid is a substance which contains more hydrogen than hydroxyl ions, so that the properties of the hydrogen ions predominate over those of the hydroxyl ions. The strong acids are electrovalent, so all the hydrogen that they contain is in ionic form and the acidic properties are marked. The weak acids are covalent, so hydrogen ions are provided only by the few molecules which dissociate and the acidic properties are less apparent than with the strong acids. Similarly an alkali is a substance which contains more hydroxyl than hydrogen ions.

The proportion of dissociation of molecules in water is constant and there is always the same ratio of hydrogen and hydroxyl ions together to undissociated water molecules. Addition or removal of ions of either type does not disturb the ratio. The effect of adding extra ions is counteracted by re-combination of some of those present into water molecules;

that of removing ions by the dissociation of more water molecules. When either of these occurs the total number of ions is maintained at the same level, but the relative concentration of the two types of ion is altered. If, for example, hydrogen ions are removed by combination with another substance, then a fall in the total number of ions is prevented by dissociation of more water molecules. This provides an equal number of hydrogen and hydroxyl ions, so the lost hydrogen ions are replaced by a mixture of hydrogen and hydroxyl ions and there are consequently more hydroxyl than hydrogen ions. Thus a fall in the hydrogen ion concentration causes a rise in the hydroxyl ion concentration. Similarly a rise in the hydrogen ion concentration causes a fall in the hydroxyl ion concentration. Altered hydroxyl ion concentration has corresponding effects on the hydrogen ion concentration.

So long as there is the same number of both types of ion the reaction is neutral, but as soon as there are more of one type than of the other the properties of the predominant ion become apparent. If the hydrogen ion concentration exceeds the hydroxyl ion concentration the reaction is acid, while if the hydroxyl ion concentration is greater than the hydrogen ion concentration the reaction is alkaline.

Behaviour of a Metal Immersed in a Solution

If a metal rod is immersed in a solution containing ions there is a tendency either for ions to pass from the metal into the solution or for ions from the solution to be deposited on the rod. The latter can occur only if ions of the same metal as the rod are present in the solution. If a zinc rod is immersed in a solution of zinc sulphate, zinc ions pass from the rod into the solution. Zinc ions are positive and electrons are left on the rod, which consequently acquires a negative charge relative to the solution. A zinc rod will also give up ions to a solution which does not contain zinc ions, such as a sulphuric acid solution. If, on the other hand a copper rod is immersed in a solution of copper sulphate, copper ions from the solution are deposited on the rod. The copper ions have a positive charge, so the rod becomes positively charged relative to the solution. Ions are deposited only if the rod is immersed in a solution which contains copper ions.

The metals can be arranged in order according to which of the above processes tends to occur, and the extent to which it occurs. The list is known as the *electrochemical series*, and a few of the substances in it are:

Potassium, sodium, zinc, hydrogen, copper, silver, platinum.

Metals above hydrogen, if immersed in a solution of standard strength, give up ions to the solution, while those below hydrogen receive their own ions from the solution, provided that these are present. In each case a potential difference is set up between the rod and the solution, the metals above hydrogen becoming negative relative to the solution, those below positive. The ionic movement continues only until a certain P.D. is established between the metal and the solution. The further the substance is from hydrogen on the list, the greater is the movement of ions and the greater the P.D. developed. Substances near the top of the list have a greater tendency to exist in ionic form than those lower down. The latter have a greater tendency to exist in atomic form. *E.g.* a hydrogen ion is neutralised to form an atom more readily than is a zinc ion, and a zinc ion is neutralised more readily than a sodium ion. Negative ions behave in a similar manner, *e.g.* a chlorine ion is neutralised more readily than a hydroxyl ion.

Passage of Current Through a Solution

Chemical effects are produced when a direct current is passed through an electrolyte, the process being known as electrolysis.

ELECTROLYTES. An electrolyte is a substance which contains ions. The molecules of the electrovalent compounds consist entirely of ions and so these substances, which provide many ions, are strong electrolytes. Those covalent compounds in which there is some dissociation of molecules provide a few ions and are weak electrolytes. In both cases the properties of the electrolyte become more apparent when the substance is dissolved in water, as there is more room for the ions to move than when it is in solid form.

The chemical changes which take place on the passage of a D.C. result in decomposition of the electrolyte. Hence the term electrolysis, which means breaking down by electricity.

The electrolysis of sodium chloride solution provides a good example of the passage of a D.C. through an electrolyte. Sodium chloride is a strong electrolyte, so when it is dissolved in water the solution contains positive sodium ions, negative chlorine ions, positive hydrogen ions, negative hydroxyl ions and water molecules (Fig. 24).

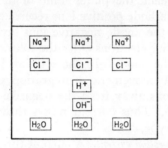

FIG. 24.—IONS IN SODIUM CHLORIDE SOLUTION.

MIGRATION OF IONS. If two metal plates are immersed in sodium chloride solution, and connected to a source of constant EMF, a current passes round the circuit. One plate receives excess electrons from the negative pole of the source of current, and is called the cathode; the other develops a defi-

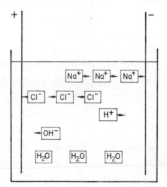

FIG. 25.—EFFECT OF CONSTANT CURRENT ON THE IONS.

ciency of electrons, being connected to the positive pole, and is called the anode. The ions are attracted more strongly to these charged plates than they are to each other, so the positive sodium and hydrogen ions move towards the negative plate, while the negative chlorine and hydroxyl ions move towards the positive plate (Fig. 25). There are therefore two streams of ions passing in opposite directions. Ions which pass towards the positive plate, or anode, are termed anions, and those which pass towards the negative plate, or cathode, are termed cations. When the ions reach the plates some of them give up their charges. At the cathode positive ions receive electrons from the electrode and at the anode negative ions give up electrons to the electrode. Thus electrons enter the solution at the cathode and leave it at the anode. In the solution between the electrodes the two way movement, or migration, of ions results in a transfer of electrons away from the negative and towards the positive electrode. Thus current passes through the solution. A current of this type, consisting of a two-way migration of ions, is known as a *convection current*. A current through the tissues of the body is a convection current, since the tissue fluids contain salts in solution and so are electrolytes.

CHEMICAL CHANGES. When ions are neutralised at the electrodes chemical changes take place.

At the cathode:
Positive sodium and hydrogen ions migrate to the cathode. Hydrogen is lower than sodium in the electrochemical series, so its ions are more easily neutralised. When hydrogen ions are neutralised, they form hydrogen gas which is given off as bubbles. The hydrogen ion concentration in the solution falls, so the hydroxyl ion concentration rises and the reaction is alkaline.

$$H^+ + e = H \qquad\qquad 2H = H_2 \uparrow$$

Hydrogen ion+electron = Hydrogen   Hydrogen gas evolved

At the anode:
Negative chlorine and hydroxyl ions migrate to the anode.

$$Cl^- - e = Cl$$
Chlorine ion — electron = Chlorine
$$Cl_2 + H_2O = HCl + HClO$$
Chlorine+Water=Hydrochloric Acid+Hypochlorous Acid

Chlorine ions give up their charge more readily than hydroxyl ions and when they are neutralised the chlorine formed reacts with the water forming hydrochloric and hypochlorous acids. Hydrochloric acid is a strong acid, providing many hydrogen ions, and so the reaction of the solution becomes acid.

If the solution is weak there may be insufficient chlorine ions. Then some of the hydroxyl ions are neutralised, forming oxygen and water. As the hydroxyl ion concentration falls the hydrogen ion concentration rises and the solution is acid in reaction.

$$OH^- - e = OH$$
Hydroxyl ion —electron=Hydroxyl
$$4OH = 2H_2O + O_2 \uparrow$$
Hydroxyl = Water+Oxygen gas evolved

These changes occur if inert electrodes are used, *i.e.* of some material, such as platinum or carbon, which is low in the electrochemical series, and so does not tend to take part in the chemical actions. If the electrodes are of materials higher in the electrochemical series they are involved in the chemical changes which are consequently somewhat different, but the details of these need not concern the physiotherapist.

The chemical changes described above occur on the passage of a direct but not an alternating current. If the current is alternating the ions move to and fro as the direction of the current changes and any acids or alkalis formed during one half cycle are neutralised when the current flows in the opposite direction.

ELECTROLYSIS OF OTHER SOLUTIONS. A similar sequence of events occurs on the passage of a direct current through other electrolytes. On application of a difference of potential the migration of ions commences. When ions reach the electrodes some of them discharge, so that electrons enter the solution at the cathode and leave it at the anode. On discharge of the ions chemical changes tend to take place. If the electrolyte contains positive ions which are lower in the electrochemical series than hydrogen, such as copper or silver, these are neutralised at the cathode in preference to the hydrogen ions. The metals so formed are deposited on the electrode, this effect being used in electroplating.

POLE TESTING. The chemical changes which occur when a D.C. is passed through an electrolyte are used in determining the polarity of a direct current source of supply. If the bare ends of two leads connected to such a supply are placed in tap-water and the current turned on, bubbles of hydrogen gas appear round the negative wire.

Alternatively litmus paper can be used. This is damped with tap-water and the bare ends of the two leads from the source of current are pressed firmly on the paper about 1 inch apart. On the passage of current blue litmus paper turns red with the acid at the anode, while red litmus paper turns blue with the alkali formed at the cathode.

THE SPEED OF MIGRATION OF IONS. The individual ions move slowly through the electrolyte, but as some are already in contact with the electrodes, current passes and chemical changes commence as soon as the EMF is applied. Ions vary considerably in size and the lighter ions move more readily and at a greater speed than the heavier ones.

NUMBER OF IONS NEUTRALISED. The number of ions neutralised at the electrodes depends on the number of electrons that enter or leave the solution, *i.e.* upon the quantity of electricity that passes. When the ions are neutralised, substances are deposited on or liberated at the electrodes, and the quantity of a substance so formed is directly proportional to the quantity of electricity that is passed. Intensity of current is the rate of flow of electrons, measured in quantity per unit time, so the amount of a substance deposited or liberated in a given time depends upon the intensity of the current. If the current is passed through a silver nitrate solution, silver is deposited at the cathode, and the weight of silver deposited in a given time depends on the intensity of the current. Hence the definition of the ampere as that intensity of current which, when passed through a solution of silver nitrate in water, deposits 0·001118 gramme of silver at the cathode in one second.

THE CONDUCTIVITY OF A SOLUTION. The greater the amount of salt dissolved in water, the better the conductivity of the solution. Ten per cent. salt solution is a better conductor than 2 per cent. because it contains more ions. The conductivity is not, however, directly proportional to the strength of the solution. In strong solutions the ions are more crowded and their migration is impeded by collisions with other ions. So, though more ions do reach the electrodes from a strong solution than a weak one, the increase is not so great as might be expected.

Production of an EMF by Chemical Action

PRINCIPLES OF CELLS. An EMF is produced by chemical action in a cell. The cell consists of two dissimilar metals immersed in an electrolyte and the principle underlying its action is the behaviour of a metal immersed in a solution, described earlier in this chapter. Metals at different points in the electrochemical series are chosen, one above and the other below hydrogen. When they are immersed in the electrolyte ions pass from one metal into the solution and this electrode becomes negatively charged. Ions from the solution are deposited on the other electrode which consequently acquires a positive charge. Thus a P.D. is set up between the metals. The ionic movement continues only until a certain P.D. is established between each metal and the solution. The voltage available from the cell is the sum of these potential differences and the EMF produced therefore depends on the position of the metals in the electrochemical series and on the electrolyte used. A particular combination of materials always provides the same EMF.

On completion of a pathway between the electrodes, outside the cell, electrons pass through this external circuit from the negative to the positive electrode. The flow of electrons tends to reduce the charge on both electrodes, but as this occurs the movement of ions within the cell recommences, maintaining the charge on the electrodes and so the P.D. between them. The negative potential of one metal and the positive potential of the other remain constant throughout, so the current obtained is direct and unvarying. The current flow is impeded not only by the resistance of the external circuit but also within the cell itself, where there is some impedance to the movement of ions. The latter is referred to as the internal resistance of the cell.

THE LECLANCHÉ CELL. There are various types of cell, the different types being made from different materials and giving different EMFs, but that in common use is the dry Leclanché cell. This consists of zinc and carbon electrodes in a

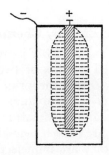

FIG. 26.—THE LECLANCHÉ CELL.

solution of ammonium chloride. The carbon replaces the second metal and is surrounded by a mixture of powdered carbon and manganese dioxide. The ionic movement within the cell results in the zinc acquiring a negative and the carbon a positive charge, the P.D. between them being 1·5 volts. In the dry Leclanché cell the zinc forms the outer case of the cell and the wire coming from it is the negative terminal. The carbon electrode is a rod in the centre of the cell and its summit forms the positive terminal (Fig. 26).

Cells in Series and in Parallel

When cells are used as a source of EMF a number are commonly connected together to form a battery. There are two ways in which the cells may be connected, in series or in parallel with each other.

Cells in Series (Fig. 27). When cells are connected in series with each other the positive terminal of the first cell is connected to the negative terminal of the second, the positive terminal of the second to the negative of the third, and so on. The external circuit is taken from the negative terminal of the first cell and the positive terminal of the last one. In this way all the current passes through each cell. Therefore the EMF of the battery is the sum of the EMFs of the individual cells, and the internal resistance of the battery is the sum of the internal resistances of the individual cells. If there are ten cells, each with an EMF of 1·5 volts and an internal resistance of 1 ohm, the EMF of the battery is 15 volts and the internal resistance 10 ohms.

Cells in Parallel (Fig. 28). When cells are connected in parallel with each other the positive terminals of all the cells are connected together and to one end of the external circuit, the negative terminals together and to the other end of the external circuit. The current passes through the external circuit from the common point where the negative terminals are connected together to the common point of junction of the positive terminals. With this arrangement the current is divided between the cells, and each portion passes through one cell only. Therefore the EMF of the battery is the same as that of a single cell. The internal resistance of the battery is, however, reduced to less than that of one cell, as when resistances are connected in parallel with each other. If the cells all have the same internal resistance, the resistance of the battery is that of one cell divided by the number of cells. Thus with a battery of ten cells, each with an EMF of 1·5 volts and an internal resistance of 1 ohm, the EMF of the battery is 1·5 volts and the internal resistance $\frac{1}{10}$ ohm.

The choice of method of connecting the cells depends on the resistance of the external circuit. If the resistance is high, a large EMF is necessary to produce an appreciable intensity of current, and the cells are connected in series with each other to provide this. There is a consequent increase in the internal resistance, but this is usually small compared with the resistance of the circuit as a whole. If the external resistance is low a small EMF is adequate to produce an appreciable intensity of current, provided that the cells themselves do not add too much

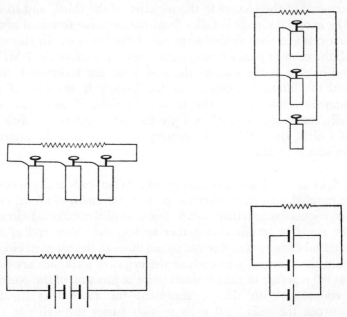

FIG. 27.—CELLS IN SERIES. LOWER DIAGRAM AS INDICATED IN CIRCUITS.

FIG. 28.—CELLS IN PARALLEL. LOWER DIAGRAM AS INDICATED IN CIRCUITS.

to the total resistance of the circuit. Consequently the cells are connected in parallel with each other in order to keep the internal resistance as low as possible. Connection of cells in parallel has the additional advantage that they last longer than if a single cell is used.

4

MAGNETISM AND METERS

Nature of Magnetism

A MAGNET is a substance showing certain properties, among which are the power of attraction for certain materials and the tendency, when free to rotate, to come to rest pointing in a north-south direction.

TYPES OF MAGNET. A type of iron ore with magnetic properties is found in certain parts of the world and this forms a *natural magnet*. The original magnets, known as lodestones, were of this material. It is possible to produce magnetic properties in certain materials which then form *artificial magnets*. Materials which can be magnetised are iron and steel and, to a lesser extent, nickel and cobalt. Soft iron readily acquires magnetic properties, but also loses these properties quickly and so forms a *temporary magnet*. Steel is considerably more difficult to magnetise but retains the properties much longer than iron, so is known as a *permanent magnet*. This term is, however, somewhat misleading as the properties are lost in time. An electric current produces magnetic effects and a coil of wire carrying a current acts as an *electromagnet*. The magnetic properties are present only so long as the current is flowing, so this is a temporary magnet.

MOLECULAR THEORY OF MAGNETISM. If a magnet is broken in two each part forms a complete magnet, however often the process is repeated. It is therefore assumed that the individual molecules of the magnetisable materials are tiny magnets. Their magnetic properties probably result from the rotation of electrons in their orbits, which constitute minute electric currents and produce the magnetic properties. When the material is not magnetised the molecular magnets lie in a haphazard manner and their magnetic properties neutralise

49

each other, but when the material is magnetised the molecules assume an orderly arrangement and their magnetic effects augment each other and become apparent (Figs. 29 and 30). In soft iron the molecules can be rearranged easily, but soon move out of their new positions so that their magnetic properties cease to be apparent. Steel is a hard metal with the molecules closely packed together, so it is more difficult to effect the rearrangement, but once it is achieved the molecules

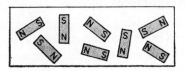
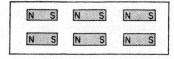

FIG. 29.—SUBSTANCE NOT   FIG. 30.—SUBSTANCE MAGNETISED.
MAGNETISED.

tend to stay in their new positions and the magnetic properties are retained. Heating or hammering a magnet accelerates the loss of magnetic properties as the increased movement of the molecules shakes them out of their orderly arrangement. The reasons that only certain materials can be magnetised is not known, but it is interesting to note that the three magnetisable elements, iron, nickel and cobalt, lie next to each other in the periodic table.

Properties of a Magnet

SETTING IN A NORTH-SOUTH DIRECTION. When a magnet is free to rotate it comes to rest with one end pointing towards the magnetic north pole of the earth, the other to the earth's magnetic south pole. The end that points north is termed the north-seeking pole, commonly abbreviated to north pole, while that which points south is called the south-seeking, or south pole. This property of a magnet is utilised in a compass, the compass needle being a small magnet.

BEHAVIOUR OF LIKE AND UNLIKE POLES. Like magnetic poles repel each other and unlike magnetic poles attract each other. If the north pole of a bar magnet is brought near to the north pole of a suspended compass needle, the latter moves away from the magnet, but if the south pole of the magnet

approaches the north pole of the compass needle this end of the
needle swings towards the magnet. The behaviour of like and
unlike poles is responsible for a magnet setting in a north-south
direction. The earth is a gigantic magnet and its magnetic
north pole has the same magnetic polarity as the south-seeking
pole of a magnet, thus it attracts the north-seeking pole of the
magnet.

TRANSMISSION OF PROPERTIES. A magnet can produce
magnetic properties in a piece of magnetisable material by
contact or by induction.

Magnetisation by contact. One method of magnetisation by
contact is to stroke a piece of iron or steel with one pole of a bar
magnet. The same pole is used throughout and the strokes are
always carried in the same direction. The end of the piece of

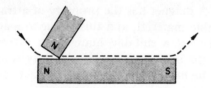

FIG. 31.—MAGNETISATION BY STROKING.

material at which the stroke commences assumes the same
magnetic polarity as the pole with which it is stroked, the end
where the stroke finishes the opposite polarity. This is in
accordance with the molecular theory of magnetism, as if the
north pole of a magnet is used it attracts the south poles of the
molecular magnets of the iron or steel and draws them towards
the point where it leaves the bar (Fig. 31).

Magnetic induction. Induction has previously been defined as
the production of magnetic or electrical properties in one
object by another without contact between them, so magnetic
induction is the production of magnetic properties in an object
by a magnet, without contact. If a piece of magnetisable
material is placed close to, but not in contact with, one pole
of a magnet, it is found to assume magnetic properties; *e.g.* a
piece of soft iron held close to a magnet will attract iron filings.
The magnetic pole attracts the unlike and repels the like poles

of the molecular magnets of the soft iron, so effecting the re-arrangement of these particles which is responsible for the magnetisation of the iron. If it is a south magnetic pole that approaches the iron, it attracts the north and repels the south

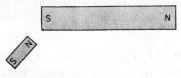

FIG. 32.—MAGNETIC INDUCTION.

poles of the molecular magnets, so setting up a north pole at the adjacent end and a south pole at the far end of the piece of iron (Fig. 32).

ATTRACTION FOR OBJECTS OF MAGNETISABLE MATERIAL. A magnet has the property of attracting objects of a magnetisable material, and this is due to magnetic induction. If a piece of a suitable material is placed near to a magnetic pole the opposite magnetic polarity is induced in its adjacent end, the unlike magnetic poles attract each other and the object moves towards the magnet.

MAGNETIC FIELD. The area around a magnet in which the magnetic forces are apparent is known as the magnetic field. The forces act along definite lines, the magnetic lines of force, which are the lines along which a free north pole would travel if it were able to move in the magnetic field. The properties of the magnetic lines of force are that they:

Travel away from the north and towards the south pole.

Tend to take the shortest pathway between two points, and so to travel in straight lines.

Tend to repel each other, as this would be the behaviour of two north poles. This may be in opposition to the pre-ceding tendency, and a balance between the two helps to determine the distribution of the magnetic field.

Travel more easily through some materials than others. The lines of force travel most easily through the magnetisable materials and the presence of such a material in the mag-netic field causes concentration of the lines of force.

The magnetic lines of force can be plotted by placing over a magnet a piece of cardboard on which iron filings are scattered. When the cardboard is tapped gently the filings arrange themselves along the magnetic lines of force. Figs. 33 and 34 show

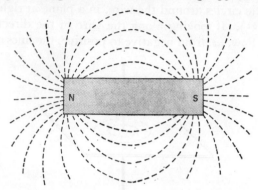

FIG. 33.—LINES OF FORCE ROUND A BAR MAGNET.

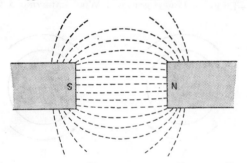

FIG. 34.—LINES OF FORCE BETWEEN OPPOSITE POLES.

the arrangement of the lines of force around a bar magnet and between unlike magnetic poles.

Magnetic Effect of an Electric Current

An electric current sets up a magnetic field around the conductor through which it is passing. This can be demonstrated by holding a wire carrying a current over and parallel to a compass needle, for as the current flows the needle is deflected to one side, indicating the presence of magnetic forces. The magnetic lines of force around a wire carrying a current can be plotted by passing a length of wire through a piece of cardboard on which iron filings are scattered. When a current is passed, and the cardboard tapped gently, the iron filings arrange themselves along the magnetic lines of force, which are found to form concentric circles around the wire, in a plane at right angles to it (Fig. 35). If looking along the wire in the direction of the electron flow, *i.e.* from negative to positive, the lines of force are

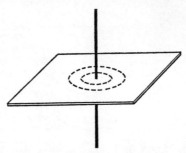

FIG. 35.—LINES OF FORCE ROUND A WIRE CARRYING A CURRENT.

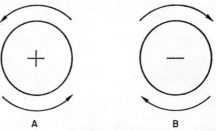

A   B

FIG. 36.—DIRECTION OF LINES OF FORCE ROUND A WIRE.
A. Looking from the negative towards the positive.
B. Looking from the positive towards the negative.

considered to move round the wire in an anticlockwise direction. If the wire is viewed from the other end, *i.e.* positive to negative, the movement will be clockwise (Fig. 36).

MAGNETIC FIELD AROUND A COIL OF WIRE. When a current is passed through a coil of wire magnetic lines of force are set up round each turn of wire and their combined effect forms a magnetic field around the whole coil. Fig. 37A shows a coil of wire through which a current is passing, Fig. 37B the same coil cut along the line SN, the lower half being seen from above. The lower turns of wire in the second diagram are viewed so that the observer is looking towards the negative end of the wire, and the lines of force rotate in a clockwise direction. The view of the upper turns is towards the positive, so the direction of the lines of force is anticlockwise. The lines of force are crowded together in the centre of the coil, but spread out at the sides and ends, emerging from one end, which forms the north pole, and returning to the other, which is the

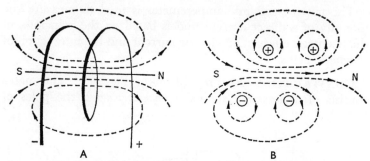

FIG. 37.—MAGNETIC FIELD AROUND A COIL OF WIRE.

south pole. Thus the magnetic poles lie at the ends of the coil and the magnetic polarity of each depends on:

1. The direction of the current flow. Reversal of the current reverses the direction of the magnetic lines of force.

2. The direction in which the coil is wound. This can be worked out with a coil wound in the opposite direction to that shown in Fig. 37.

There are various rules for determining the magnetic polarity of a coil, a simple one being Ampère's rule:

Imagine a man swimming with the electron flow (negative to positive) and facing the centre of the coil, the north pole is on his right.

Many of the rules for determining magnetic polarity assume the current flow to be from positive to negative. This must always be considered when using the rules, as tracing the current incorrectly for the particular rule gives the wrong magnetic polarity.

ELECTROMAGNETS. An electromagnet consists of a coil

of wire wound on a soft iron bar. When a current passes through the coil a magnetic field is set up and the soft iron core is magnetised by induction, so that its field is added to that produced by the current. Thus a strong magnetic field is formed, which can be turned on and off as required by starting and stopping the current flow. Soft iron is chosen for the core because it is easily magnetised and demagnetised.

The Moving-coil Milliamperemeter

The moving-coil milliamperemeter is used to measure the intensity of a direct current and is based on the principles of the magnetic effect of an electric current and the interaction of magnetic fields.

CONSTRUCTION OF THE METER (Fig. 38). The meter consists of a horseshoe-shaped *permanent magnet*, the poles of

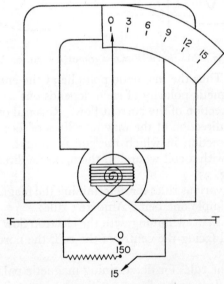

FIG. 38.—THE MILLIAMPEREMETER.

which are extended by pole pieces and lie close together, providing a concentrated magnetic field. The pole pieces are hollowed out to receive the solenoid and iron core which lie between them. The *iron core* is a circular piece of soft iron, fixed to the casing of the meter, which serves further to concentrate the magnetic field. The *solenoid* is a coil of fine, insulated, copper wire wound on a light frame of non-magnetisable metal. The frame is on a pivot which passes through a hole in the iron core, so that the solenoid is free to rotate around the stationary core. The coil is wound in such a way that when it is at rest the turns of wire lie parallel to the lines of force of the magnet. A *pointer* is attached to the frame of the solenoid and moves over a *scale* which is usually marked, in one direction only, up to 15 or 25 milliamperes. Some meters have a scale which reads in both directions, the zero point being in the centre. A *hairspring* lies in front of the solenoid frame and has one end attached to the frame, the other to a fixed point. The direction in which it is wound is such that it tightens as the solenoid rotates, so resisting the movement. If the meter has a scale which reads in both directions there are two hair-springs, wound in opposite directions so that each resists movement in one direction. The hair-springs also serve to lead the current to and from the solenoid. *Shunt circuits* are provided, which can be included in parallel to the solenoid when required. Their arrangement and purpose are explained below.

WORKING OF THE METER. Current passes from one terminal, through the hair-spring and solenoid and out by the other terminal. As the current flows through the solenoid a magnetic field is set up, the poles being at the ends of the coil. The north pole of the solenoid is attracted by the south pole and repelled by the north pole of the permanent magnet, and the south pole is influenced in a corresponding manner. The solenoid therefore swings round, carrying the pointer over the scale. The rotation is resisted by the hair-spring, which controls the movement and keeps it steady, and the amount of rotation depends on the strength of the magnetic field around the solenoid and therefore on the intensity of the current that passes. When the current ceases to flow the solenoid is no longer an electromagnet and the hair-spring brings it and the pointer back to the zero position. The direction in which the solenoid rotates depends on the direction of the current, as reversal of the current changes the magnetic polarity of the solenoid. So if the scale is marked to one side only the current must always be passed through the meter in the same direction.

The meter is suitable only for the measurement of a direct current. If an alternating current were passed the magnetic polarity of the solenoid would change continually, too rapidly for movement to take place. If the D.C. is varied in intensity, as when it is surged or interrupted, the solenoid swings to and fro and damage to the hair-spring would result if the meter were kept in the circuit for more than a short time.

THE SHUNT CIRCUITS. These may be included in the circuit if required. When no shunt circuit is included, as with the selector switch on the point marked 15 in Fig. 38, all the current passes through the solenoid and the intensity is shown on the scale. If a larger intensity of current is to be passed the selector switch is moved to include a shunt circuit. This is usually a "10" shunt, marked with ten times the maximum number shown on the scale (150 in Fig. 38), and with a resistance of one-ninth of that of the solenoid. When the shunt circuit is included some current passes through this circuit and some through the solenoid. In accordance with Ohm's law, the intensity of current in each pathway is inversely proportional to the resistance, so the current in the shunt pathway is nine times that in the solenoid. Thus for every one milliampere that passes through the solenoid nine pass through the shunt circuit, making a total of ten in the meter as a whole. The total current passing through the meter is ten times that in the solenoid, and as it is the latter which is registered on the scale, the reading shown must be multiplied by ten. The scales of some meters are marked with two sets of figures, to indicate the readings with and without the shunt circuit included. Alternatively a small o may be placed after each of the figures to show the reading when the ten shunt is included.

Thus the provision of shunt circuits increases the range of intensities of current that can be measured. In order to measure small intensities accurately the solenoid must be light and delicately made. The passage of currents of large intensity might burn out the fine wire, but the diversion of a known proportion of the current through the parallel pathway makes it possible to measure currents of large intensity without damage to the solenoid.

An additional pathway of extremely low resistance is usually provided and is included in the circuit by moving the selector switch to the point marked o or off; the solenoid may at the same time be cut out of the circuit. The resistance of this pathway is negligible compared with that of the solenoid, so virtually all the current passes through it, none through the solenoid, and there is no deflection of the pointer. This shunt is included when a surged or interrupted current is used, in order to avoid damage to the hair-spring from continual movement of the solenoid.

WIRING INTO THE CIRCUIT. When resistances are wired in series with each other the intensity of current is the same in all parts of the circuit, so the milliamperemeter is placed in series with the other components in which the intensity of current is to be measured. The addition of resistances in series in a circuit increases the total resistance and so reduces the intensity of the current. Therefore the resistance of the meter is kept as low as possible in order to minimise this effect.

CARE OF THE METER. Care must be taken not to pass a current of too great an intensity, so that the needle is forced beyond the end of the scale. This would strain the hair-spring, the needle would not return exactly to the zero position and readings would be inaccurate. The hair-spring may also be strained by the pointer swinging to and fro when an interrupted or surged current is used, but this can be avoided by inclusion of the o shunt.

The Voltmeter

CONSTRUCTION AND WORKING (Fig. 39). A voltmeter is used to measure the potential difference between two points. It is similar in construction to the moving coil milliamperemeter, except that a large resistance is placed in series with the solenoid, giving the meter as a whole a definite known resistance.

According to Ohm's law $I = \dfrac{E}{R}$, so if the total resistance of the meter is 1,000 ohms a potential difference of one volt between the terminals will produce a current of one milliampere. The point to which the needle is deflected by this current is marked 1 volt. Similarly a potential difference of 2 volts will produce a current of 2 milliamperes, and the scale is marked accordingly. Alternatively, if the total resistance is 8,000 ohms a P.D. of 1 volt will produce a current of $\frac{1}{8}$ milliampere and 8 volts will be required to produce 1 milliampere. So the point to which the needle is deflected by 1

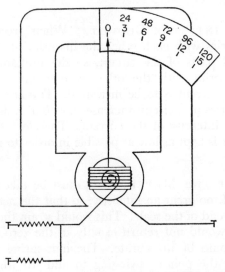

FIG. 39.—THE VOLTMETER.

milliampere is marked 8 volts, that to which it is deflected by 2 milliamperes 16 volts, etc. Thus the point to which the needle is deflected by a certain intensity of current is marked with the number of volts that must have been applied to produce that current in the particular resistance.

Many voltmeters are provided with alternative resistances to allow a greater range of EMFs to be measured. A short, insulated wire connected to the top of the meter is usually the negative terminal, while a prong forms the positive terminal. Where there is more than one resistance a separate prong, and usually separate scale markings, are provided for each. The scale reads one way only, so it is important that the current is passed through the meter in the correct direction.

WIRING INTO THE CIRCUIT. The purpose of a voltmeter is to measure the potential difference between two points, so it is connected to these two points in parallel to any other circuit that may exist between them. This is because the P.D. across all circuits in parallel to each other is the same. The addition of parallel pathways to a circuit causes a decrease in the resistance and an increase in the total intensity of current,

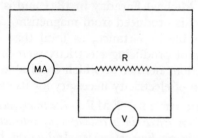

FIG. 40.—CONNECTION OF MILLIAMPEREMETER
AND VOLTMETER INTO A CIRCUIT.

especially if the resistance of the additional pathway is low. Therefore the voltmeter has a high resistance, otherwise its inclusion would cause a marked increase in the total intensity of current in the circuit. Fig. 40 shows the connection of a milliamperemeter and a voltmeter into a circuit to measure the intensity of current in, and P.D. across, the resistance R.

Meters for Measuring Alternating Currents

The moving-coil meter is suitable for use only with D.C., so to measure the intensity of an A.C. a meter of a different type must be employed. Such meters are rarely encountered in electromedical apparatus. A meter is not necessary in the apparatus supplying a low-frequency A.C. and with a high-frequency A.C. it is usual to convert the current passing through the meter into D.C. and use a moving-coil meter, as this is more accurate and robust than other types.

5

ELECTROMAGNETIC INDUCTION

Principles of Electromagnetic Induction

ELECTROMAGNETIC induction was first demonstrated by Michael Faraday in 1831 and is the means by which electricity is produced from magnetism. The discovery was of considerable importance, as until that time the only known methods of producing electricity were by friction and by chemical action, neither of which is suitable for the large-scale production of electricity necessary for its extensive use.

PRODUCTION OF THE EMF. *Electromagnetic induction is the production of an EMF in a conductor by interaction between the conductor and magnetic lines of force.* Induction has previously been defined as the production of electrical or magnetic properties in one object by another without contact between them, electrostatic and magnetic induction being examples. Electromagnetic induction is the production of electrical properties in one object, which must be a conductor of electricity, by the magnetic lines of force surrounding another object. The two objects do not come in contact with each other, but it is necessary for one to move relative to the other, as it is only when magnetic lines of force cut across the conductor, or the conductor across the lines of force, that the EMF is produced. Thus the essentials for electromagnetic induction are:

A conductor.
Magnetic lines of force.
Movement of one of these relative to the other.

If the conductor forms part of a closed circuit a current flows when the EMF is induced.

The production of an EMF by electromagnetic induction can be illustrated by three simple experiments, which were originally carried out by Michael Faraday:

Experiment 1. A coil of wire is connected to a milliampere-meter to form a closed circuit (Fig. 41). A bar magnet is thrust into the coil, allowed to remain stationary for a moment and then withdrawn. Deflection of the needle of the meter is observed when the magnet is entering and leaving the coil, but when the magnet is stationary the needle returns to zero. The coil of wire is the conductor and the bar magnet provides the magnetic lines of force. When the magnet is moved relative to the coil the magnetic lines of force cut across the turns of wire, an EMF is produced and current flows in the circuit, causing deflection of the needle of the meter. When the

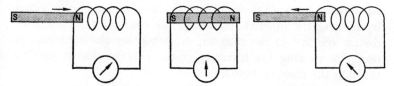

FIG. 41.—EXPERIMENT TO ILLUSTRATE ELECTROMAGNETIC INDUCTION.

magnet is stationary there is no movement of the lines of force relative to the coil and no EMF is induced. Movement of the coil of wire over the stationary magnet produces the same results, as when the coil is moved it cuts the magnetic lines of force.

Experiment 2. The preceding experiment is repeated using an electromagnet instead of a bar magnet. A direct current is passed through the electromagnet and sets up magnetic lines of force which, as the electromagnet is moved in and out of the coil, cut the turns of wire and induce EMFs in them. As in the preceding experiment, deflection of the needle of the meter is observed only when the electromagnet or the coil is moved.

Experiment 3. The same apparatus is used as for the preceding experiment, but the electromagnet, which is known as the primary coil, remains stationary within the coil connected to the meter. The latter is known as the secondary coil. An interrupted D.C. is passed through the electromagnet and deflection of the needle of the meter is observed when this current increases or decreases in intensity, but not when it is flowing at constant strength. When the current in the electro-magnet increases in intensity magnetic lines of force spread out around this coil, cutting the secondary coil and inducing an EMF in it. When the current in the primary coil is of constant intensity the magnetic field remains steady, so the lines of force are not cutting across the secondary coil and no EMF is produced. When the current in the electromagnet decreases in intensity the magnetic field collapses and the lines of force again cut the secondary coil, inducing an EMF in it.

Thus the conductor in which the EMF is induced is usually a coil of wire, while the magnetic lines of force may be supplied either by a permanent magnet or by an electromagnet. Movement of one of these relative to the other may be provided by moving the magnet relative to the conductor, or the conductor relative to the magnet, or, when an electromagnet is used, by varying the intensity of the current that is passing through the electromagnet.

DIRECTION OF THE INDUCED EMF. In the first and second of the experiments described above the milliampere-meter needle swings in one direction when the magnet enters the coil, the other way when it is withdrawn. In the third experiment the needle swings one way when the primary current is increasing in intensity, the other way when it is

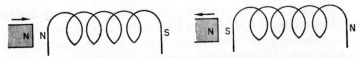

FIG. 42.—MAGNETIC POLARITY RESULTING FROM INDUCED CURRENTS.

decreasing. The direction of the deflection of the needle depends on the direction of the induced current, so it is apparent that there is some connection between the direction of the induced EMF and that of the movement which produces it.

Lenz's law states that *the direction of the induced EMF is such that it tends to oppose the force producing it.* When the north pole of a bar magnet approaches a coil of wire, the direction of the induced EMF is such that the current it produces sets up a magnetic field with the north pole at the end of the coil to which the north pole of the magnet is approaching. Like magnetic poles repel each other, so the approach of the magnet is opposed. When the magnet is withdrawn the direction of the current is such that a south pole is set up at the end of the coil from which the north pole of the magnet is removed, attracting the magnet and so opposing the movement. This is shown in Fig. 42. Using a primary and secondary coil, with a varying current flowing in the primary, when the current in the primary coil is rising in intensity the EMF induced in the secondary coil is in the opposite direction to that applied to the primary, so tending to produce a current in the opposite direction to the primary current. When the primary current is falling in intensity the EMF induced in the secondary coil is in the same direction as that applied to the primary, so tending to produce a current in the same direction as that which was flowing in the primary.

STRENGTH OF THE INDUCED EMF. *Faraday's Law* of electromagnetic induction states that *the strength of the induced EMF is proportional to the rate of change of the magnetic field.* When moving a bar magnet relative to a coil of wire, as in the first experiment, the deflection of the milliamperemeter needle is increased if the magnet is moved more quickly or if a stronger magnet is used. The latter increases the number of lines of force which cut the coil in a given time, so in both cases the rate of change of the magnetic field is increased and a greater EMF induced. When using primary and secondary coils, the rate of change of the magnetic field depends on the rate at which the primary current varies in intensity. The more rapid the variation in the intensity of this current the greater is the induced EMF.

The strength of the induced EMF is proportional to the inductance of the conductor in which it is produced. Inductance is the ability of the conductor to have an EMF induced in it. It depends primarily on the number of turns of wire present in the coil, but also on the proximity of the turns of wire to each other and whether or not there is an iron core present to concentrate the magnetic field. Inductance is a constant factor for any particular conductor and is measured in Henries. *A Henry is the*

D

inductance of a conductor in which an EMF of one volt is induced by a current varying at the rate of one ampere per second.

In all three of the experiments described a greater deflection of the needle of the meter is observed if the number of turns of wire in the secondary coil is increased, provided that the rate of change of the magnetic field remains constant.

MUTUAL INDUCTION. When an EMF is induced in one conductor by the magnetic field set up by a varying current flowing in another conductor the process is known as mutual induction. The third of the experiments described above is an example of mutual induction.

SELF-INDUCTION. When a current flows through a coil of wire it sets up magnetic lines of force around each turn of wire. If the current varies in intensity these lines of force spread

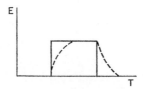

FIG. 43.—EFFECT OF SELF-INDUCTION.

out and collapse as the current intensity increases and decreases. The moving lines of force cut across turns of wire adjacent to the one from which they are set up and induce EMFs in them. Thus a varying current flowing in a conductor induces an EMF in that same conductor, the process being known as self-induction. The effects of the self-induced EMF can be determined by applying the laws of electromagnetic induction.

The direction of the induced EMF, like that induced in the secondary coil, is in accordance with Lenz's Law. Thus when the applied current is rising in intensity the induced EMF is in the opposite direction to the applied EMF. This "back" EMF opposes the increase of the intensity of current and makes it more gradual. When the applied current is falling in intensity the induced EMF is in the same direction as the applied EMF. This "forward" EMF prolongs the flow of current and makes the fall more gradual. This is shown in Fig. 43. The continuous line indicates the EMF applied, the dotted line the current which is obtained.

As with mutual induction, the strength of the induced EMF is proportional to the inductance of the conductor and to the rate of change of the magnetic field, the latter depending on the rate of change of the current flowing in the conductor. The greater the rate of change of this current the greater is the speed at which the magnetic lines of force cut neighbouring turns of the coil, and so the greater the EMF induced. For this reason high-frequency currents, which alternate at the rate of one million times a second or more, set up a greater self-induced EMF than the alternating main current, which only alternates fifty times per second, while a constant direct current only produces a self-induced EMF when it is switched on and off.

INDUCTIVE REACTANCE. The "back" EMF produced by self-induction opposes the rise in intensity of current. Thus it impedes the flow of current in the circuit and may prevent it from reaching as great an intensity as it would otherwise have done. This impedance, resulting from the self-induced EMF, is known as inductive reactance. The amount of impedance from inductive reactance depends on the strength of the self-induced EMF which is determined by:

1. The inductance of the conductor, with which it varies directly.
2. The rate of change in intensity of the current flowing in the conductor. The greater the rate of change the greater is the self-induced EMF. Thus there is no inductive reactance with a constant D.C., but it is present whenever the current varies in intensity, and increases as the frequency increases.

EDDY CURRENTS. Any conductor lying within a varying magnetic field has an EMF induced in it. If the conductor consists of a solid piece of material the EMF gives rise to circular currents at right angles to the magnetic lines of force. These currents are greatest near the surface of the conductor and are known as eddy currents. They are liable to be set up in, for example, the soft iron core of an electromagnet through the coil of which a varying current is flowing. The eddy currents are often undesirable as they tend to reduce the magnetic effect of the current by setting up a magnetic field in opposition to the original one. To prevent their occurrence conductors which must lie within varying magnetic fields are laminated, *i.e.* split into strips, which are often insulated from each other by thin layers of varnish. The strips lie at right-angles to the direction in which the currents would flow, electrons are unable to pass from one strip to the next and so the currents are prevented.

Principles of the Dynamo

The dynamo is used for the production of an EMF by electromagnetic induction. A coil of wire lies between the poles of a magnet and some means of rotating the coil is provided. Various sources of power may be used for this purpose, such as water power, a steam engine or some type of motor. As the coil rotates the turns of wire cut across the magnetic lines of force and the essentials for electromagnetic induction are present, *i.e.* there is movement of a conductor relative to magnetic lines of force. Thus an EMF is induced in the coil of wire. As the coil rotates the turns of wire cut the magnetic lines of force first in one direction, then in the other, so the current produced is alternating. A collecting device is used to convey the current from the moving coil of wire to the external circuit. This may transmit the alternating current directly to the circuit or may change into a direct current. Thus the dynamo can be constructed to supply either A.C. or D.C. It is the apparatus used for all large-scale production of electricity, including that for the main supply.

The Static Transformer

The static transformer is based on the principles of electromagnetic induction and is used to alter the voltage of an alternating current and to render the current earth-free.

CONSTRUCTION OF THE TRANSFORMER. The trans-
former consists of two coils of insulated wire, the primary and
secondary coils, wound on a laminated soft iron frame. The
coils are completely insulated from each other and one usually
contains more turns of wire than the other. The frame is often
rectangular in shape and the coils may be wound on opposite
bars of the frame or one on top of the other on a central bar
(Fig. 44).

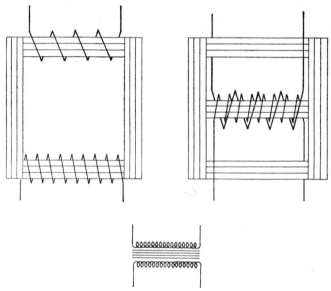

FIG. 44.—CONSTRUCTION AND SYMBOL. STATIC TRANSFORMER.

WORKING OF THE TRANSFORMER. An alternating current is passed through the primary coil and sets up a varying
magnetic field which cuts the secondary coil and induces an
EMF in it. It is essential that the primary current varies in
intensity, otherwise there is no movement of the magnetic field
relative to the conductor and no EMF is induced in the secondary coil. There is no electrical connection between the
primary and secondary coils, the energy being transmitted

from one to the other by electromagnetic induction. The core
serves to concentrate the magnetic field. It is made of soft iron
because this material is easily magnetised and demagnetised.
It is laminated to prevent eddy currents.

FUNCTIONS OF THE TRANSFORMER. The two principal
functions of the transformer are:

1. To render the current earth-free. The electricity supplied
from the mains is an earthed current. The current is produced
in the power station by a dynamo and is distributed to the consumer by two cables, the live and neutral wires. One of the
output terminals of the source of supply is connected to earth
and the distribution cable which is taken from this terminal is
connected to earth at intervals along its course. This is the
neutral wire (N in Fig. 45) and it is always at zero potential.

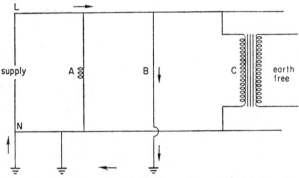

FIG. 45.—EARTHED AND EARTH FREE CURRENT.

The live wire (L in Fig. 45) is taken from the other output
terminal of the supply. It is insulated from earth and is
electrically charged. When current is required, a circuit is
completed between the two cables and so between the two
supply terminals (A in Fig. 45). If, however, a connection is
inadvertently made between the live cable and earth (B in
Fig. 45) this also completes a circuit between the output
terminals, the earth forming part of the conducting pathway.
Current in this circuit is shown by the arrows in Fig. 45. Thus
any connection between the live wire and earth completes a

circuit through which current flows. Should some person form part of this circuit he receives an "earth" shock.

The danger of earth shock is reduced by the use of a static transformer. The main current is passed through the primary coil (C in Fig. 45) and induces an EMF in the secondary coil. So long as there is no electrical connection between the primary and secondary coils, the latter has no connection to earth. Thus if a connection is inadvertently made between the secondary circuit and earth it does not complete a circuit, no current passes to earth and there is no danger of earth shock. The earth does not form any part of the conducting pathway of the secondary current, which is said to be earth-free. The transformer renders the current earth-free only so long as there is no electrical connection between the primary and secondary coils. Should the insulation between the coils break down the secondary circuit would be connected to earth and there would be a danger of earth shock. For this reason all transformers supplying current for the treatment of patients must be constructed in a way which makes such an occurrence impossible.

2. To alter the voltage of an alternating current. The EMF induced in the secondary coil is proportional to the number of turns of wire in this coil. If there are more turns of wire in the secondary than in the primary coil, the EMF obtained from the secondary is greater than that applied to the primary. This is known as a step-up transformer. *E.g.* if there are twice as many turns of wire in the secondary as in the primary coil and an EMF of 100 volts is applied to the primary, 200 volts will be induced in the secondary. If there are fewer turns of wire in the secondary than in the primary coil the EMF induced in the secondary is less than that applied to the primary, and the device is known as a step-down transformer. *E.g.* if the primary has four times as many turns of wire as the secondary and an EMF of 100 volts is applied to the primary, 25 volts will be induced in the secondary coil. If there are the same number of turns of wire in both coils the EMF induced in the secondary is the same as that applied to the primary. This is known as an even-ratio transformer, and its sole function is to render the current earth-free.

CURRENT OUTPUT. Although the EMF can be altered

it is impossible to obtain from the secondary circuit a greater amount of electric power, *i.e.* a greater number of watts, than is supplied to the primary circuit. An increase in the EMF is accompanied by a corresponding decrease in the intensity of current available, while reduction of the EMF increases the available intensity of current. If an EMF of 100 volts is supplied to the primary coil and produces a current of 10 amperes, the power is 1,000 watts. If the secondary coil has ten times as many turns of wire as the primary, the EMF induced in it will be 1,000 volts, but as 1,000 watts is the maximum power available the intensity of the current in the secondary circuit cannot exceed 1 ampere. If, however, the secondary coil has one-tenth the number of turns of wire of the primary, the EMF is reduced to 10 volts and the maximum intensity of current available increased to 100 amperes. Actually the intensity of current that can be obtained is rather less than that given above, as there is some loss of energy in the transformer.

The above figures represent the maximum intensity of current that can be obtained. Provided that it does not exceed this amount, the actual intensity depends on the EMF and the resistance of the circuit. For example, if 1,000 watts are available and the EMF is 100 volts, the maximum current is 10 amperes. If the resistance of the external circuit is 50 ohms, then by Ohm's law:

$$I = \frac{E}{R} = \frac{100}{50} = 2 \text{ amperes}$$

This is less than the maximum available and a current of 2 amperes flows in the external circuit. If, however, the resistance of the external circuit is 5 ohms, then by Ohm's law:

$$I = \frac{E}{R} = \frac{100}{5} = 20 \text{ amperes}$$

The maximum current available is, however, only 10 amperes, so a current of 10 amperes flows in the external circuit.

When the resistance of the external circuit is high it is an advantage to step up the voltage, as a large EMF is necessary to produce an appreciable current. The intensity of the current in the high resistance will in any case be low, so it is unimportant that the maximum that is available is reduced. When the external circuit has a low resistance it is an advantage to step down the voltage. A small EMF is adequate to produce an appreciable current and it is desirable that a large intensity of current should be available if it is required.

NATURE OF THE SECONDARY CURRENT. The type of current induced in the secondary coil can be deduced by the application of Lenz's and Faraday's laws of electromagnetic induction. Graphs of the primary current and secondary EMF are shown in Fig. 46. When the primary current is rising

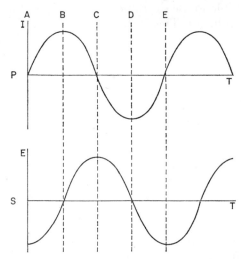

FIG. 46.—PRIMARY CURRENT AND SECONDARY EMF
IN A TRANSFORMER.

in intensity, the EMF induced in the secondary coil is in the opposite direction to that applied to the primary (AB and CD), while when the primary current is falling in intensity the EMF induced in the secondary coil is in the same direction as that applied to the primary (BC and DE). The intensity of the primary current rises at first quickly, then more slowly, so the magnetic field increases at first quickly, then more slowly. Therefore the EMF induced in the secondary is at first strong but becomes weaker (AB and CD). When the primary current is at its maximum there is an instant when the current intensity, and so the magnetic field, is not changing, and so the EMF in the secondary coil is at zero (B and D). When the intensity of the primary current falls, it does so at first slowly, then more quickly, so the secondary EMF is at first weak, getting stronger (BC and DE). The graphs show that the secondary current is similar to that in the primary coil, but a quarter of a cycle behind it.

VARIABLE TRANSFORMERS. Tappings may be provided so that either the primary or secondary coil can be varied in length. By varying the number of turns of wire in the primary coil it is possible to use the same piece of apparatus on supplies of different voltages. This is shown in Fig. 47. The higher the

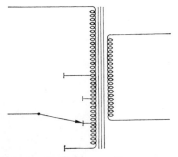

FIG. 47.—A VARIABLE TRANSFORMER.

voltage of the supply the more turns of wire are included in the primary coil, and the EMF induced in the secondary is kept constant. This device is included in many modern pieces of apparatus, and care should be taken to see that the control is in the right position for the supply used. Connection to a 200 volt supply with the selector switch on 100 volts would result in the passage of a current of considerable intensity, as only a small part of the coil is included, and this would probably burn out the transformer windings.

Variation in the length of one of the coils may also provide a way of controlling the power supplied to the apparatus. One method of increasing the output of a short wave diathermic machine is by reducing the number of turns of wire included in the primary coil of the transformer. When this is done the ratio of turns of wire in the secondary coil to that in the primary is increased and so the EMF induced in the secondary is increased.

Tappings may be taken from different points on the secondary coil to supply different voltages to separate circuits in the same piece of apparatus, or one transformer may have several secondary coils. This will be observed in many of the circuits in which valves are used.

AUTOTRANSFORMER. The autotransformer consists of a single coil of insulated wire wound over a laminated iron core. In Fig. 48 it is tapped at two points, C and D. When used as a step-up transformer the coil between C and D acts as the

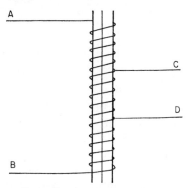

FIG. 48.—AUTOTRANSFORMER.

primary and the whole coil as the secondary. For a step-down transformer the whole coil is the primary, and the part between C and D the secondary. The EMF and current output of the secondary depend, as in other transformers, on the relative number of turns of wire in the part between C and D and the whole coil. The autotransformer has certain disadvantages. It can only be used for a small step up or down in voltage and it does not make the current in the secondary earth-free.

The Choke Coil

A choke coil is included in a circuit in order to produce a self-induced EMF.

LOW-FREQUENCY CHOKE COIL. This consists of many turns of insulated wire wound on a laminated soft iron frame, usually on the central bar of a rectangular frame (Fig. 49). When a current which is varying in intensity is passed through the coil, magnetic lines of force are set up which cut the turns of wire and induce EMFs in them. There are many turns of wire so the coil has a considerable inductance and the self-induced EMF is large. The core serves to concentrate the magnetic field; it is made of soft iron so that it is easily magnetised and demagnetised and is laminated to prevent eddy currents.

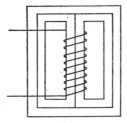

FIG. 49.—CHOKE COIL.

HIGH-FREQUENCY CHOKE COIL. A high-frequency current varies very rapidly in intensity so tends to produce a considerable self-induced EMF. Consequently it is unnecessary to have a great many turns of wire in a high-frequency choke coil, or to wind them on a soft iron core. The coil usually consists of several turns of insulated wire wound on a bobbin of some non-conducting material.

USES OF THE CHOKE COIL. The self-induced EMF which is set up when a varying current is passed through a choke coil retards the rise of current to maximum and prolongs the current flow when the intensity is falling. This tends to even out the variations in the intensity of the current, which is one of the purposes for which a choke coil is used.

When a high-frequency current is passed through a choke coil the inductive reactance is considerable, so the coil may be used to impede the flow of such a current. The impedance offered to a low-frequency or direct current is considerably less than to a high-frequency current, and a choke coil may be included in a circuit to prevent the flow of a high-frequency current but at the same time allow the passage of one of lower frequency.

6

THE CONDENSER

Potential and Capacity

ELECTRICAL potential is the electrical condition of a body due to the stored-up energy of its electric charge. It gives rise to certain properties which the object does not possess in its neutral state, among which is a repelling power for a like charge. Electrical potential is measured in volts, but it is often convenient to consider it in terms of one of the properties, *i.e.* the greater the potential the greater is the repelling power for a like charge. The electrical potential of a body depends on the quantity of electricity with which it is charged, the greater the quantity, the greater being the electrical potential. It also depends on the capacity of the object, which is its ability to hold an electric charge and is determined by the material and surface area of the object. The greater the capacity the less is the potential produced by a given quantity of electricity. Thus the electrical potential of a charged body varies directly with the quantity of electricity with which it is charged and inversely with its capacity, *i.e.*:

$$E = \frac{Q}{C} \text{ where } E = \text{potential measured in volts.}$$

Q = quantity of charge measured in coulombs.

C = capacity measured in farads.

Principles of the Condenser

A condenser is a device for storing an electric charge and is based on the principles of static electricity.

If a charged conductor is brought close to, but not in contact with, another conductor, its capacity is increased, especially if the other conductor bears the opposite electric charge. When the objects approach each other the charges concentrate on the adjacent surfaces and the electric field, which exists around any charged object, is concentrated between them (Fig. 50). This reduces the repelling power of the objects for a like charge, that is, their electrical potential is reduced. The quantity of electricity with which the objects are charged is unaltered and

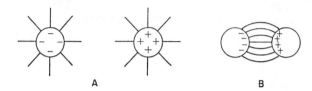

A   B

FIG. 50.—ELECTRIC FIELDS AROUND CHARGED CONDUCTORS.

so to effect the reduction in potential their capacity must be increased. The capacity is increased because energy is stored in the insulating material which separates the charged bodies. The electrons in the atoms of an insulator are strongly attracted by the central nuclei and so cannot easily be dislodged from their orbits. When the conductors are charged the electrons in the insulating material are attracted by the positive and repelled by the negative charge, and although they are unable

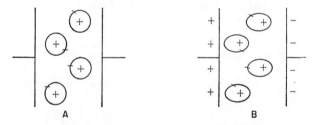

A   B

FIG. 51.—DISTORTION OF ELECTRON ORBITS.

to leave the atoms their orbits are drawn to one side and the molecules distorted (Fig. 51). So long as the conductors are charged the molecules of the insulating material remain distorted and consequently in a state of strain, like a stretched spring. As soon as the distorting force is removed the molecules return to their original formation, releasing energy as they do so. Thus when two conductors are placed adjacent to each other, but separated by an insulator, their capacity is increased. This is the basis of a condenser, which in its simplest form consists of two metal plates separated by an insulator, which is called the dielectric.

DISPLACEMENT CURRENTS. When the plates of a condenser are charged there is a momentary movement of electrons within the atoms of the dielectric as molecular distortion takes place. When the plates are discharged the molecules return to their original form and again there is a movement of electrons within the atoms. This electron movement is known as a displacement current and occurs only in an insulator, where the electrons are too strongly held by the central nuclei for them to leave the atoms. Any change in the charge on the plates of a condenser is accompanied by a displacement current in the dielectric.

Capacity of a Condenser

The capacity of a condenser is its ability to hold an electric charge.

MEASUREMENT OF CAPACITY. The capacity of a condenser, like that of a conductor, is measured in farads. One *farad* is the *capacity of a condenser which is charged to a potential difference of one volt by one coulomb of electricity*. The practical unit is the microfarad, which is 1/1,000,000 of a farad.

The potential difference between the plates of a charged condenser depends on:

1. The quantity of electricity with which the condenser is charged. The greater the quantity of electricity the greater is the P.D.

2. The capacity of the condenser. If the condenser has a large capacity a certain quantity of electricity does not produce so great a P.D. as if the capacity is small, in which case the charge is more concentrated. Consequently a condenser of large capacity requires a greater quantity of electricity to produce a certain P.D. between the plates than would be necessary for one with a small capacity.

Thus the potential difference between the plates of a charged condenser varies directly with the quantity of electricity with which it is charged and inversely with its capacity, *i.e.*:

$$E = \frac{Q}{C}$$ where E = potential difference measured in volts.

Q = quantity of electricity measured in coulombs.

C = capacity measured in farads.

The condenser consists of two conductors, and so it is the potential difference between them that must be considered, otherwise the above factors correspond to those which determine the potential of a charged conductor. The capacity of a conductor is assessed by the potential produced by a given quantity of electricity, that of a condenser by the potential difference.

FACTORS DETERMINING CAPACITY. The capacity of a condenser depends on:

The surface area of the plates.
The material of the plates.
The width of the dielectric.
The material of the dielectric.

As with a single conductor, a large surface area of plates results in a large capacity. Some materials hold the electric charge more readily than others, and if the plates are of such a material the condenser has a large capacity.

If the dielectric is narrow there is a strong force of attraction between the opposite charges on each side of it. Consequently the charges are very concentrated on the adjacent surfaces of the plates, there is a strong electric field between them and marked distortion of the molecules of the dielectric. Thus much energy is stored and the condenser has a large capacity.

The material of the dielectric also affects the capacity, as molecular distortion occurs more readily in some materials than others, and these are capable of storing a greater amount of energy. The effect of a material on the capacity of a condenser is indicated by its *dielectric constant*. This is *the ratio of the capacity of a condenser with the material as the dielectric to the capacity of a similar condenser with dry air as the dielectric.* Dry air is taken as having a dielectric constant of 1, so if a material has a dielectric constant of 5 it is capable of storing five times as much energy as dry air, and a condenser with this material as the dielectric has five times the capacity of an otherwise similar condenser with dry air as the dielectric. The dielectric constant of mica is 5, glass 4 or 10 (depending on the type), oil and paraffin wax about 2.

Dielectric constant must not be confused with dielectric strength, which is the power of the material to resist the tendency for electrons to pass through it. The electrons would pass in the form of a spark, from the negative to the positive plate, if a sufficiently high difference of potential were applied.

Construction of a Condenser

A condenser consists essentially of two conductors separated by a dielectric, and the simplest form of condenser is made up of two flat metal plates with a sheet of insulating material between. Flat plates are used to provide a large surface area, and in order that the condenser may be compact each plate usually consists of several sheets of metal which are connected together and to one terminal. The metal sheets are placed alternately with those of the other plate, from which they are separated by layers of insulation (Fig. 52, left hand diagram).

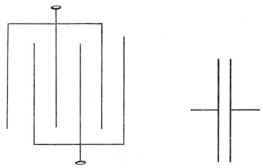

FIG. 52.—SYMBOLS FOR CONDENSERS.
Left: large capacity.   Right: small capacity.

The plates are of copper, aluminium or tinfoil, the dielectric of glass, mica or paper impregnated with paraffin wax. For condensers of tinfoil and paraffin wax paper an alternative construction may be adopted, the plates and dielectric consisting of long strips of the materials which are rolled up like a scroll.

THE VARIABLE CONDENSER. This is a condenser of which the capacity can be varied and which usually consists of aluminium plates with air as the dielectric. Each plate is commonly made up of several sheets of metal which are semicircular in shape and are interleaved with those of the other plate, from which they are separated by gaps containing air. One plate is fixed while the other can be rotated by a knob so that the metal sheets move in or out between those of the fixed plate (Fig. 53). When the metal sheets of one plate are lying

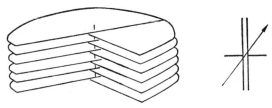

FIG. 53.—THE VARIABLE CONDENSER.
CONSTRUCTION AND SYMBOL.

between those of the other, the capacity is at a maximum, but as one is moved from within the other the effective surface area, and so the capacity, is reduced. Such condensers are used for tuning a wireless set and also a short-wave diathermic machine.

Electric Field

An electric field exists between the plates of a charged condenser, the forces acting along electric lines of force. Characteristics of these are given in Chapter 1 and determine the distribution of the condenser field; the relevant points are:

(1) The lines of force tend to take the shortest pathway between two points, but, in opposition to this, behave as if they repel each other. The balance between these two tendencies is partly determined by the distance between the condenser plates. If the plates are widely separated much energy is

expended in passing from one plate to the other and little is available for the lines of force to repel each other, but if the plates are close together the repulsion is more marked and the field spreads (Fig. 54). The spread is especially marked at the

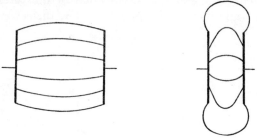

Fig. 54.—ELECTRIC FIELDS BETWEEN PLATES
OF CONDENSERS.

edges of the field where there are few lines of force to limit the outward bending (Fig. 55).

(2) The lines of force pass more easily through some materials than others. They travel easily through materials of high dielectric constant, less readily through those of low dielectric constant. If the material between the plates is of low dielectric constant it offers considerable impedance to the lines of force, the effect is the same as that of wide separation of the plates and there is little spread of the electric field. Material of

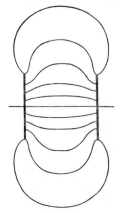

Fig. 55.—SPREAD OF AN ELECTRIC FIELD.

high dielectric constant allows the lines of force to pass easily and the field spreads as when the plates are close together. A small area of a material of high or low dielectric constant affects the distribution of the lines of force. A small area of high dielectric constant causes concentration of the lines of force (Fig. 56), while they avoid an area of low dielectric constant (Fig. 57).

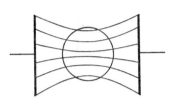
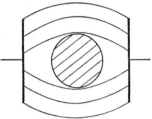

FIG. 56.—EFFECT OF MATERIAL OF HIGH DIELECTRIC CONSTANT.

FIG. 57.—EFFECT OF MATERIAL OF LOW DIELECTRIC CONSTANT.

Charging and Discharging a Condenser

CHARGING A CONDENSER. A condenser can be charged directly or by electrostatic induction. To charge by electrostatic induction one plate is connected to a source of supply, so that it acquires a positive or negative charge, and the other to earth. The sequence of events by which the earthed plate is charged is described under electrostatic induction in Chapter 1. More usually the condenser is charged directly by connecting the two plates to the opposite poles of a source of supply. Electrons pass from the negative pole on to one plate, which becomes negatively charged, and from the other plate to the positive pole, leaving this plate with a positive charge. As the movement of electrons takes place a current flows in the circuit and a difference of potential is set up between the plates.

When the condenser is first connected to the source of supply the plates are uncharged and there is no opposition to the movement of electrons on to one plate and off the other, but as the plates become charged a P.D. is set up between them, which acts in the opposite direction to that of the source of supply. This reduces the effect of the latter and causes a fall in the intensity of current. At first, when the intensity of current is great, the charge builds up rapidly and so the intensity of current falls rapidly. When the intensity of current becomes less the charge builds up more slowly and the intensity of current falls slowly. When the difference of potential between the plates is equal to that of the source of supply there are two equal and opposite forces, no further movement of electrons takes place and the current ceases. The graph of this current is shown in Fig. 58.

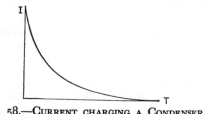

FIG. 58.—CURRENT CHARGING A CONDENSER.

If the condenser has a large capacity a greater quantity of electricity is required to charge it to the same potential difference as the source of supply than if it has a small capacity, and so it takes longer to charge. Thus the time required to charge the condenser varies directly with its capacity.

When the condenser is charged it can be disconnected from the source of supply and the charge is retained.

DISCHARGE OF A CONDENSER. When a circuit is completed between the plates of a charged condenser electrons flow from the negative to the positive plate until the charges are neutralised. As the condenser discharges, the potential difference between the plates becomes less and so the intensity of current falls. At first, when the difference of potential between the plates is high, the intensity of current is great and the condenser discharges rapidly. As the potential difference falls the intensity of current is reduced and the discharge becomes less rapid. The graph of this discharge current is similar to that shown in Fig. 58.

DURATION OF THE CONDENSER DISCHARGE. The duration of the condenser discharge depends on:

The capacity of the condenser.

The resistance of the circuit through which the condenser discharges.

A condenser of large capacity, when charged to a certain P.D., contains a greater quantity of electricity than one of small capacity which is charged to the same P.D. If the two condensers are connected to identical circuits it takes longer for the larger one to discharge than for the smaller, as there is a greater quantity of electricity to pass through the circuit. Thus the duration of the discharge varies directly with the capacity of the condenser.

If the ohmic resistance of the pathway between the condenser plates is high, the current which flows is of small intensity. The condenser therefore takes longer to discharge than if the ohmic resistance of the circuit is low, in which case a current of greater intensity is obtained. Thus the duration of the discharge varies directly with the resistance of the circuit.

Duration of condenser discharge varies with $C \times R$.

Where C=capacity of condenser measured in farads.

R=resistance of the circuit measured in ohms.

The terms "long" and "short" used with reference to the condenser discharges are only comparative as, unless the capacity and resistance are very large, the discharge only takes a fraction of a second.

CONDENSER DISCHARGE THROUGH AN INDUCTANCE. If the condenser is discharged through a circuit of low ohmic resistance containing an inductance, the electrons flow from one plate to the other and back again, passing forwards and backwards several times with diminishing force until the current dies

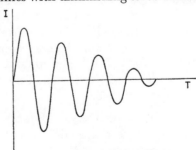

FIG. 59.—OSCILLATING CONDENSER DISCHARGE.

away. This is called an oscillating discharge and the graph of the current is shown in Fig. 59. The frequency of the oscillations may be very high, often several million cycles per second.

The oscillation of the current is due to the self-induced EMF which is set up in the inductance as the current varies in intensity. The self-induced EMF retards the rise of current and prolongs the flow when the intensity is falling. So when the excess electrons from the negative plate have passed through the circuit to the positive one and both plates are at the same potential, the electron movement continues. This recharges the condenser with reversed polarity, as the plate which was previously positive acquires excess electrons and that which was originally negative is left with a deficiency. When the self-induced EMF dies away the condenser discharges again, producing a flow of current in the opposite direction to the original one, and the process continues. The amplitude of each flow of current is less than that of the preceding one, as there is some loss of energy in the circuit. This type of discharge is obtained only in a circuit of low ohmic resistance. If the resistance is high the intensity of current is low and its rate of change is not great enough to produce an appreciable self-induced EMF. Consequently the condenser is not recharged after the first flow of current and no oscillations are produced. The oscillating discharge, including the factors which determine the frequency of the current, is considered fully in Chapter 17.

CAPACITIVE REACTANCE. As a condenser is charged the potential difference developed between the plates offers an increasing impedance to the charging current. If the condenser has a large capacity a greater quantity of electricity is required to charge it to the same potential difference as the source of supply than if it has a small capacity, so the impedance does not develop so quickly.

When a condenser is connected to a source of D.C., it charges until the potential difference between the plates is equal to that of the source of supply, then blocks any further flow of current. If, however, the source of supply is A.C. the condenser charges and discharges as the current alternates. When the alternations are of low frequency the condenser still offers considerable impedance to the current flow, as there is ample time for the charge to build up on the plates before the direction of the applied current changes. If, however, the frequency is increased, the direction of the current changes before the P.D. between the condenser plates is equal to that of the source of supply. The more frequent the change in direction the less is the P.D. developed between the plates and the less the impedance to the electron flow. This may be compared to water moving in a pipe divided by some elastic partition (Fig. 60). If a pump is applied acting in one direction, the partition stretches to its limit, then blocks the flow of water. If the pump acts first in one direction, then the other, the water and partition move to and fro as the direction changes. If this

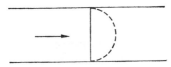

FIG. 60.—TO ILLUSTRATE CAPACITIVE RESISTANCE.

occurs infrequently considerable impedance to the flow of water is encountered, but if the frequency is increased the direction changes before the partition has stretched to its limit, and so the impedance to the flow is much reduced.

This impedance offered to the flow of current by a condenser in the circuit is known as capacitive reactance and the amount of capacitive reactance depends on:

The capacity of the condenser, with which it varies inversely.
The frequency of the current, as the higher the frequency the less is the impedance.

USES OF CONDENSERS. Condensers are used for various purposes in electromedical apparatus. The following being some examples:

(1) To make the current more comfortable for the patient in the Smart-Bristow faradic coil (Chapter 11).

(2) To reduce the variations in the intensity of a rectified current (Chapter 7).

(3) To control the timing of electronic interrupters and surgers (Chapter 10).

(4) To produce a high-frequency current (Chapter 18).

7

VALVES AND SEMICONDUCTORS

The Thermionic Valve

A VALVE is a device which transmits in one direction only, common examples being the valves of the veins and heart and that of a bicycle tyre. A thermionic valve is a device which transmits an electric current in one direction only, and the term thermionic implies that heat plays some part in the working. There are various types of thermionic valve, which are named according to the number of electrodes that they contain.

THE DIODE VALVE. This is the simplest form of thermionic valve and contains two electrodes, the filament and the plate, which are enclosed in an evacuated glass bulb. For a current to pass across the valve the filament must be heated and a P.D. applied so that the plate is positive in relation to the filament. When the filament is heated thermionic emission (page 271) takes place and electrons are freed from the wire. If a P.D. is then applied so that the plate is positive in relation to the filament, the free electrons are attracted through the vacuum to the plate and current passes across the valve. No current flows if the filament is cold, as no electrons are liberated, nor if the P.D. is reversed so that the plate is negative relative to the filament, as there are no free electrons in the region of the plate. Thus electrons can pass from the filament to the plate, but not in the reverse direction, and the valve transmits current in one direction only.

The intensity of the current that flows across the valve depends on the heating of the filament and on the P.D. between the filament and the plate. Increasing the former increases the number of electrons that are liberated and an increase in the

P.D. makes available a greater force to attract them across the valve. The filament is heated by passing an electric current through it, and the circuit which carries this current is known as the filament circuit. The circuit which carries the current which passes across the valve is termed the plate or anode circuit (Fig. 61).

The filament may be of the directly or indirectly heated type. The former consists of loops of fine wire made of thoriated

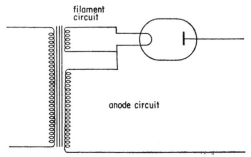

FIG. 61.—FILAMENT AND ANODE CIRCUITS.

tungsten. Tungsten is used because it tolerates the repeated heating and cooling and it is impregnated with thorium oxide, or some similar substance, as this material allows thermionic emission to take place at a fairly low temperature. The loops of wire are supported on hooks, with small springs which take up the slack when the wire expands. The indirectly heated filament also consists of fine loops of wire through which the heating current is passed, but these are embedded in insulating material and the whole surrounded by a metal cylinder from which the thermionic emission takes place and which acts as the cathode of the valve. The anode plate is of some metal which does not readily allow thermionic emission and is in the form of a cylinder surrounding the filament or cathode. There are three pins on the base of the valve, two connected to the filament and one to the plate. The pins fit into suitable sockets and are unevenly spaced so that the valve cannot be inserted into the circuit incorrectly. The valve may be evacuated or contain an inert gas at a low pressure. The pressure inside the glass bulb must be low so that there is minimal impedance to the electron movement. If a gas is introduced it must be one that will not take part in chemical changes when the valve is hot. The construction and symbols for a diode valve are shown in Fig. 62.

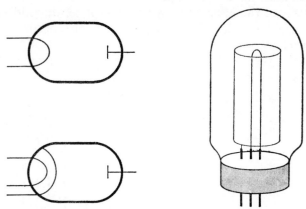

FIG. 62.—THE DIODE VALVE SYMBOLS AND CONSTRUCTION.
Symbols: Upper—with directly heated filament;
Lower—with indirectly heated cathode

THE TRIODE VALVE. This is constructed in a similar manner to the diode, but in addition contains a third electrode, the grid, which is placed between the filament and the plate (Figs. 63 and 64). The grid, which surrounds the filament, may consist of a metal cylinder perforated like a sieve to allow the electrons to pass through, or, more usually, may be a spiral of metal wire. A lead from the grid is brought to a pin outside the base of the valve, so there are four pins, two for the filament, one for the grid, and one for the anode.

When the filament is heated a current can be passed through the valve, as in the diode, in one direction only, *i.e.* from the filament to the plate. If the grid is uncharged it has no effect on the current, as the electrons pass through the openings in it and on to the anode. If the grid is charged negatively from some outside source, it repels electrons so that the current is reduced in intensity or, with a stronger charge, stopped completely. If, however, the grid is charged positively the electrons can pass and the current flows. The intensity of the current is then greater than when the grid is uncharged, as the positive charge on the grid, as well as that on the anode, is attracting electrons away from the filament. Most of these pass through the grid and on to the anode. The charges applied to the grid from an external source are known as grid bias and, as the grid lies closer to the filament than does the plate, the grid charge has a greater influence on the flow of current than has a similar charge on the anode.

The strength of the current flowing across the valve can be regulated, as in the diode, by altering the temperature of the

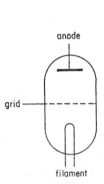

Fig. 63.—Triode Valve.
Symbol

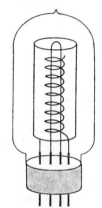

Fig. 64.—Triode Valve.
Construction

filament or by altering the positive charge applied to the anode. In addition, the flow of current across the triode valve can be regulated by adjusting the bias of the grid.

The triode valve has various functions in electromedical apparatus, the principal ones being its use for the production of the interrupted direct and other muscle stimulating currents and, in conjunction with a condenser and an inductance, for the production of high-frequency currents. It is not used specifically as a rectifier, but will always rectify the current that passes through it.

Semiconductors

PRINCIPLES. A conductor of electricity is a material, usually a metal, in which there are free electrons which readily move to constitute an electric current. An insulator is a material in which the electrons are firmly held, either by their central nuclei or by forming bonds with other atoms to build up the crystalline structure, so that they are not free to move. A semiconductor is a material which permits current flow in some circumstances. In germanium, for example, thermal agitation of the molecules can free some of the electrons from their bonds and render the material capable of transmitting current.

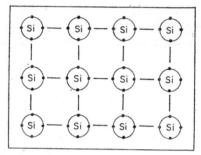

Fig. 65.—Atoms in a Crystal of Silicon.

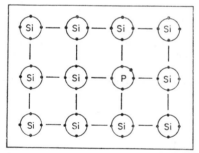

Fig. 66.—n–Type Semiconductor. Phosphorus Introduced into Silicon.

This is termed an intrinsic semiconductor. Other materials become capable of transmitting current when a small amount of another substance is introduced into them. Such a material is termed an impurity semiconductor, and silicon provides an example.

An atom of silicon has four electrons in its outer shell, and in a crystal of silicon these are held in forming bonds with neighbouring atoms, so that there are none free to transmit an electric current (Fig. 65). Introduction of some other material can, however, render silicon capable of conducting. A phosphorus atom has five electrons in its outer shell, so if some phosphorus atoms are introduced among the silicon atoms, each phosphorus atom has one electron that is not held in a bond with other atoms (Fig. 66). Thus there are free electrons and the material is capable of conducting a current by a movement of electrons in the same way as a metallic conductor. Such a material is termed an *n-type semiconductor*. An aluminium atom has three electrons in its outer shell, so if some aluminium atoms are introduced among the silicon atoms there are not enough

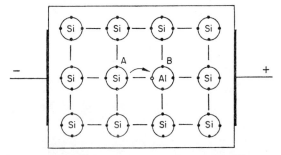

FIG. 67.—P–TYPE SEMICONDUCTOR. PASSAGE OF CURRENT
THROUGH SILICON CONTAINING ALUMINIUM.

electrons to form the bonds and some unoccupied bonds, or "holes," are left. If a P.D. is applied to such a material, electrons move from some of the atoms into unoccupied bonds nearer to the positive pole, so that as the electrons move away from the negative towards the positive, the unoccupied bonds, or "positive holes," move from the positive towards the negative pole. In Fig. 67 one electron from atom A moves into the hole in atom B, leaving a hole in A, so that the hole has moved from B to A. The movement of positive holes from the positive towards the negative is equivalent to a movement of electrons from negative to positive and constitutes an electric current. A material which transmits current in this way is termed a *p-type semiconductor*.

CONTACT BETWEEN SEMICONDUCTORS. When an n-type semiconductor, which has free electrons, is placed in contact with a p-type semiconductor, which has positive holes, electrons move from the former to occupy holes in the latter, while positive holes move in the reverse direction. Both were originally electrically neutral, so the transfer of electrons sets up a P.D. at the junction, the n-type semiconductor acquiring a positive charge and the p-type semiconductor a negative charge. The transfer of electrons continues until a certain P.D is established, then this prevents any further electron movement.

CONDUCTION ACROSS SEMICONDUCTOR JUNCTION. When the semiconductors are connected to a source of EMF, the P.D. at their junction affects the flow of current. If the n-type semiconductor is made more negative than the equili-

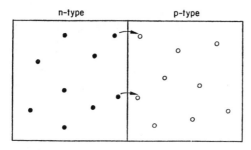

FIG. 68.—MOVEMENT OF ELECTRONS BETWEEN SEMICONDUCTORS.

brium value and the p-type more positive, electrons lost from the former are replaced from the supply, while excess electrons are withdrawn from the latter to the supply. The P.D. at the junction is reduced, electrons are able to pass from the n-type to the p-type semiconductor and current flows in the circuit. If, however, the p-type semiconductor is made negative relative to the n-type, the P.D. at the junction opposes the electron movement and no current can flow until the applied P.D. reaches a certain critical value. Therefore current can pass more easily in one direction than in the other, and the device constitutes a semiconductor diode.

METAL RECTIFIERS. A metal rectifier works on the same principle as the semiconductor diode, and one type consists of a copper disc coated on one surface with copper oxide. Copper oxide is a p-type semiconductor and copper, being a metal, has free electrons, so acts like an n-type semiconductor. Thus when the two materials are in contact a P.D. is set up at their junction. When the rectifier is connected into a circuit with the copper negative relative to the copper oxide, current passes much more easily than when the polarity is reversed. In the latter case no current flows until the EMF exceeds 8 volts. A series of discs can be used to rectify larger voltages, but must be separated from each other by suitable materials, otherwise the P.D.s developed at the contacts would cancel each other out.

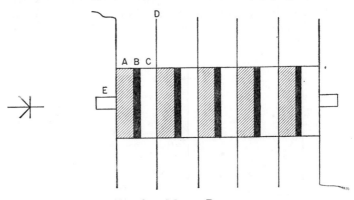

FIG. 69.—METAL RECTIFIERS.
A. Copper disc. B. Copper oxide coating and layer of graphite.
C. Lead disc. D. Cooling fin. E. Insulated rod.

The rectifier consists of an appropriate number of copper discs, which have been oxidised on one surface, mounted on an insulated rod. In contact with the copper oxide is a layer of graphite, then a lead disc and an aluminium cooling fin separates it from the next unit. The materials are chosen so that a P.D. develops only at that surface of the copper oxide which is in contact with the copper. Lead discs are used to separate the rectifying units because, being a soft metal, it makes good contact with the other discs when they are bolted together. The cooling fins serve to radiate the heat generated, which would otherwise interfere with the working, and are also used to lead the current in and out of the rectifier. The construction and symbol for the rectifiers are shown in Fig. 69. In the symbol the arrow head represents the copper, *i.e.* shows the direction of electron flow.

Selenium rectifiers are also used. Selenium is a p-type semiconductor and a tin alloy in contact with it acts as the n-type. The rectifying units are separated by appropriate materials and each will rectify up to 18 volts.

TRANSISTORS. A transistor consists of two thick layers of one type of semiconductor, termed the emitter and the collector, separated by a thin layer of the other type of semiconductor,

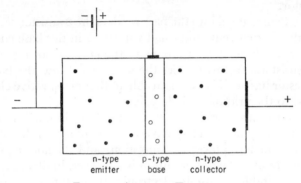

FIG. 70.—AN N–P–N TRANSISTOR.

termed the base. In a p-n-p transistor the emitter and the collector are of p-type, the base of n-type semiconductor, while in the n-p-n transistor the position of the materials is reversed. The latter is the type of transistor described below. As soon as contact is made between the materials, P.D.s develop at their junctions. In an n-p-n transistor the emitter and the collector are of n-type semiconductor so both become positive relative to the p-type base. If the device is then connected to a source of EMF with the emitter negative and the collector positive, no current flows unless the EMF exceeds the critical value. Electrons could cross the emitter-base junction but are unable to pass from the base to the collector, as the movement is opposed by the junction P.D.

When, however, a second source of EMF is connected to the base and the emitter, with the base positive relative to the emitter the transistor becomes capable of transmitting current.

E

Electrons can cross from the negative n-type emitter to the positive p-type base, so current flows in this emitter-base circuit. In this circuit there is a thick layer of n-type semiconductor, a thin layer of the p-type, so the current consists largely of a movement of electrons, and electrons from the emitter soon pass into the base. The base now has an adequate supply of electrons, and as it is very thin these come close to the base-collector junction and are attracted into the collector to replace those that had migrated into the base. This reduces the barrier effect at the base-collector junction and current flows across the transistor.

Thus a current fed into the base renders the transistor capable of conducting current, and small variations in this base current produce much greater variations in the current flowing across the transistor. In this respect the current fed into the base of a transistor has an effect comparable to that of a positive charge applied to the grid of a triode valve.

Transistors are used in preference to valves in much modern electrical equipment. They have the advantages of durability, long life and low power consumption, and do not require a heating circuit. The power output is, however, limited, so while they are suitable for use in electronic stimulators they are not as yet generally used to replace the valves of short-wave diathermic machines.

Rectification of Alternating Current

Rectification is the conversion of alternating current into direct current and the two types of rectifier used in electro-medical apparatus are the diode valve and the metal rectifier.

HALF-WAVE RECTIFICATION. If one valve or metal rectifier is included in the circuit, current can pass in one direction only and the flow is blocked during alternate half-cycles of alternating current. This is shown in Fig. 71, where the continuous line represents the current which flows, the dotted line the reverse waves which are obliterated. The resulting current is unidirectional, pulsating and interrupted and the process by which it is obtained is termed half-wave rectification. A current of this type would flow in the anode

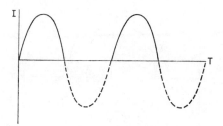

FIG. 71.—HALF-WAVE RECTIFICATION.

circuit in Fig. 61 and a similar circuit using metal rectifiers is shown in Fig. 72. In this diagram XY is the secondary coil of the transformer supplying the apparatus. When current flows through the primary coil an EMF is induced in XY, and this EMF is applied to the output circuit.

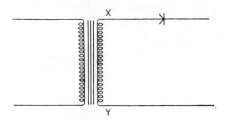

FIG. 72.—ARRANGEMENT FOR HALF-WAVE RECTIFICATION.

When X is negative and Y positive electrons pass from X through the rectifier and output circuit back to Y. When Y is negative and X positive no current flows because it is unable to cross the rectifier.

FULL-WAVE RECTIFICATION. The arrangement of the circuit can be such that the direction of the current is reversed during alternate half-cycles of A.C. Fig. 73 shows the resulting current, which is represented by the continuous line. The dotted line shows the alternate half-cycles before reversal. The current obtained is unidirectional and pulsating, but not interrupted, and the process by which it is obtained is termed

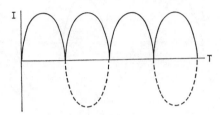

FIG. 73.—FULL WAVE RECTIFICATION.

full-wave rectification. Examples of circuits which produce full-wave rectification are:

(1) VOLTAGE-HALVING CIRCUIT. A rectifier is connected to each end of the secondary coil of the transformer. Both rectifiers are arranged to allow current to pass in the same direction, and both are connected to the same lead to the output circuit. The centre of the secondary coil is connected to the other lead. This is shown in Fig. 74. When the direction of the A.C. is such that X is negative and Y positive, electrons

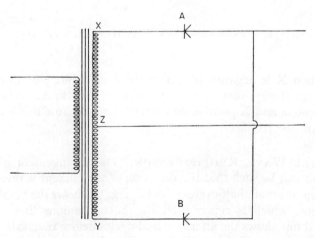

FIG. 74.—VOLTAGE HALVING CIRCUIT USING METAL RECTIFIERS.

cannot pass into the circuit from X because they cannot cross the rectifier A. The point Z is midway between X and Y, so is at zero potential. Consequently it is more negative than Y and electrons pass from Z through the external circuit and back by rectifier B to Y. When X is positive and Y negative electrons still pass from Z through the external circuit in the same direction as before, returning via rectifier A to X. Only half of the secondary coil of the transformer is used during each half cycle of A.C., so the EMF supplied to the output circuit is half of that which is induced in the coil.

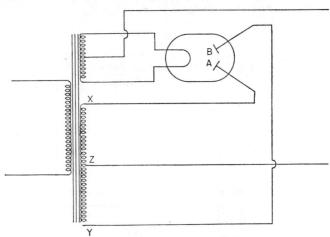

FIG. 75.—VOLTAGE HALVING CIRCUIT USING A VALVE.

A diode valve with two anode plates can be used in a similar circuit and is connected as shown in Fig. 75. Current passes as in the preceding circuit. When X is negative and Y positive current cannot flow round the circuit from X as it is unable to cross the valve in this direction. It therefore flows from Z round the external circuit to the filament of the valve, across the valve to anode B, which is positive in relation to the filament, and back to Y. When X is positive and Y negative current flows from Z through the external circuit to the filament and back via anode A to X.

(2) THE WESTINGHOUSE BRIDGE. Four blocks of recti-

fiers are used, connected as shown in Figs. 76 and 77. Fig. 76 is the usual method of drawing the circuit. The rectifiers are shown in a diamond arrangement, the input wires being connected to opposite corners of the diamond and the output wires taken from the other two corners. Two rectifiers (A and

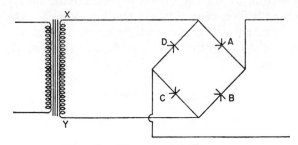

FIG. 76.—WESTINGHOUSE BRIDGE.

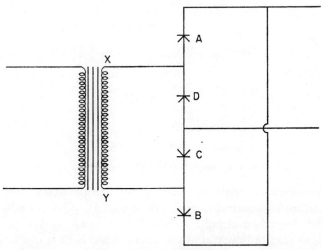

FIG. 77.—WESTINGHOUSE BRIDGE.

B) are directed towards one output wire, the other two (C and D) away from the second output wire. In the apparatus the rectifiers will be seen to form one straight block with connections taken at intervals along it. This arrangement is shown in Fig. 77, and is basically the same as that in the preceding diagram.

When the direction of the A.C. is such that X is negative
and Y is positive, current passes from X through rectifier A
to the output circuit, rectifiers B and D preventing it from
taking any other pathway. The current returns from the output
circuit, then passes through rectifier C, the only route back to
Y, the positive end of the transformer coil. When X is positive
and Y negative current passes from Y through rectifier B,
round the output circuit and back by rectifier D to X. Thus
the current always passes in the same direction through the
output circuit, and full wave rectification is obtained. There
is some drop in voltage owing to the resistance of the rectifiers,
but this is much less than that which occurs in the voltage
halving circuit.

SMOOTHING CIRCUIT (Fig. 78). The current obtained
from the rectifying circuit is unidirectional but varies considerably in intensity. In order to eliminate these variations
and render the current suitable for application to a patient a
smoothing circuit is used. This consists of one or two condensers
wired in parallel to the output circuit and a choke coil in series
with this circuit.

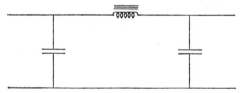

FIG. 78.—SMOOTHING CIRCUIT.

When the EMF of the rectified current rises, current flows in
the external circuit and at the same time the condensers are
charged. When the EMF falls the intensity of the current in the
output circuit falls, but the condensers discharge round this
circuit and augment the current flow so that the intensity does
not fall to zero. Thus the variations in the intensity of current
are reduced. The condensers have a large capacity so that they
offer little impedance to the charging current and hold a

considerable quantity of electricity to discharge round the circuit.

As the current varies in intensity a self-induced EMF is set up in the choke coil. When the intensity of the current is rising the self-induced EMF opposes the applied EMF and retards the rise of current. When the intensity of the current is falling the self-induced EMF is in the same direction as the applied EMF and prolongs the current flow. These effects further reduce the variations in the intensity of the current.

The current obtained from the smoothing circuit varies slightly in intensity but is suitable for use for constant D.C. treatments.

8

MAIN SUPPLY

PRODUCTION. Currents for main supply are produced by means of dynamos at the power stations. The essential principle of the dynamo is that an EMF is induced by the movement of a conductor and a magnetic field in relation to each other. Mechanical energy must be available to provide the movement. Water power is cheap and satisfactory for this purpose where it is available, but other forms of power are frequently used, such as oil or steam engines. Fuel is necessary to operate the latter, and nuclear energy is increasingly used for this purpose.

TYPE OF CURRENT. Dynamos can be constructed to produce either A.C. or D.C. When electricity was first produced for main distribution the latter was preferred, but now it has in most districts been replaced by A.C., which has a number of advantages. The construction of the dynamo is such that a greater voltage can be produced with A.C. than with D.C.; also the possibility of altering the voltage of A.C. with static transformers makes it more suitable than D.C. for long distance transmission. When the current is to be carried for long distances the EMF is stepped up to several thousand volts (e.g. 132,000 volts for the standard grid, 275,000 volts for the super-grid) with a corresponding reduction in the intensity of current. This low intensity current can be carried by comparatively thin cables, which cost less than the thick ones required for currents of large intensities. Over long distances there is a certain loss in voltage, but with the very high EMFs used this is only a small proportion of the total, and the original level can be restored by passing the current through a step-up transformer. The ease of transmission makes it possible to supply country districts at a reasonable cost and in addition to these advantages in production and distribution, the construction of much modern apparatus is such that it works only on an A.C. supply.

DISTRIBUTION. As explained in the section on static transformers, distribution is by means of one live wire and one neutral wire which is connected to earth. This method of distribution is much cheaper than if two live wires were used, as only one of the cables needs to be insulated, but the current is not earth-free. The cables may be carried across country by pylons or, in towns, taken underground enclosed in thick layers of insulation.

THE GRID SYSTEM. This is a system by which the electricity supplies throughout the greater part of the country are linked together. The supply is A.C. at 240 volts and a frequency of 50 cycles per second. A three-phase current is used. Each dynamo has three coils of wire which follow each other through the magnetic field so that a separate current is generated in each coil. One end of each coil is connected to a live distribution line while the other ends are connected together and to earth. Distribution of current is by three live cables, one from each of the dynamo coils, and one neutral cable, which is common to the three live wires. These can be observed on the pylons which carry the cables across country. The current from the power stations is fed into a system of high tension cables extending through the country. Where a district

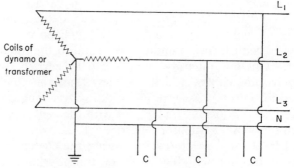

FIG. 79.—DISTRIBUTION OF ELECTRIC POWER.

is to be supplied the cables are tapped and the voltage stepped down at a transformer station. One end of each of the secondary coils of the transformer is connected to earth, and distribution throughout the area is again by three live wires and one neutral wire. Each consumer receives one of the live wires and the neutral wire (Fig. 79). As the current is alternating, the live wire is alternately negative and positive, the neutral wire being at zero potential throughout.

The grid system has the advantages that all areas supplied receive the same voltage and type of current, large demands in one area do not put an excessive load on any particular power station, and breakdown of one power station does not cut off the supply to any area. It is not necessary for all the generators to be in operation all the time, so maintenance work is facilitated and the amount of stand-by equipment can be reduced.

Wiring of Houses

DISTRIBUTION IN HOUSE (Fig. 80). The current gener-ated in the power station is supplied to the consumer by one live wire and one neutral wire, so the current is not earth-free. The current, on entering the house, passes through the main fuses and the meter, which are the property of the supply authority and should not be tampered with by the occupier. Next comes the main switch, which can be employed to cut off the current supply to the house, and the house main fuses, then the various circuits are taken in parallel to each other. This method of wiring is adopted so that each circuit receives the full voltage of the supply, the current in each is unaffected by that in the others and they can be used independently of each other. Switches and fuses are wired in series with the supply points.

LIGHT AND POWER CIRCUITS. The circuits in the house can be divided into two categories, the light and power circuits. The light circuits have a 5 ampere fuse for each 4 to 6 light points, and the wiring is designed to carry a slightly larger intensity of current than the fuses. The power circuits may be arranged in various ways:

(1) Similar to the light circuits but with stronger wiring and a fuse for each supply point (Fig. 80). Thirteen ampere fuses

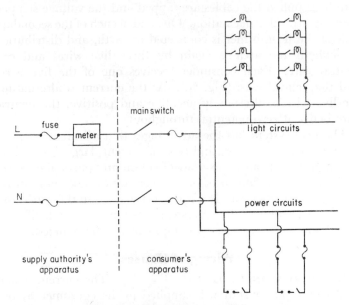

FIG. 80.—DISTRIBUTION IN HOUSE.

are used in modern wiring, 15 ampere fuses in that of older construction, and the cables can carry a slightly larger intensity of current than the fuses.

(2) A ring main may be used (Fig. 81). A complete loop is taken from each of the two supply cables and supply points are wired in parallel with each other between the loops. Fused plugs are used, so no fuses are incorporated in the wiring of the individual points, but a 30 ampere fuse is placed on the live wire entering the ring. This cable carries current from both sides of the loop, that is, from two wires, each of which can carry at least 15 amperes, hence the high rating of the fuse. Spurs may be wired in parallel to the supply points (S in Fig. 81), but both the number of spurs and the area that may be covered by the ring are limited by regulations, so in a large building there may be several rings, each with its own 30 ampere fuse.

(3) In addition to either of the above, subcircuits may be used for different installations, such as an electric cooker or

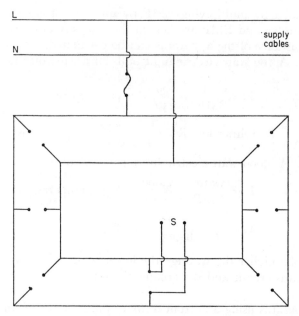

FIG. 81.—THE RING MAIN.

immersion heater or, in the Physiotherapy Department, for certain equipment, such as apparatus which uses a particularly large intensity of current.

(4) In some cases the light and power circuits divide immediately on entering the building and separate meters are provided, this method being used if different rates are charged for light and power. A similar method is employed if some of the electricity is supplied at off-peak rates. The circuits receiving this current have their own meter and a timing clock which limits their use to times when other demands are at a minimum.

The actual intensity of the current that flows in each circuit is determined by the apparatus that is connected to it. The intensity of the current depends on the EMF and the resistance, and the EMF is constant, being determined by the source of supply. Therefore the intensity of the current depends on the resistance, with which it varies inversely. All apparatus is marked with the voltage of the supply for which it is designed and the wattage that it uses on that supply. Wattage is calculated by multiplying EMF by intensity of current, so if the wattage and EMF are known the intensity of current and the resistance of the apparatus can be calculated.

E.g. A 100 watt electric light bulb for a 240 volt main.

$$I = \frac{\text{watts}}{\text{EMF}} = \frac{100}{240} = 0 \cdot 417 \text{ ampere.}$$

By Ohm's law $R = \dfrac{E}{I} = \dfrac{240}{0 \cdot 417} = 576 \text{ ohms.}$

E.g. A 2,000 watt electric fire for a 240 volt main.

$$I = \frac{\text{watts}}{\text{EMF}} = \frac{2,000}{240} = 8 \cdot 333 \text{ amperes.}$$

$$R = \frac{E}{I} = \frac{240}{8 \cdot 333} = 28 \cdot 889 \text{ ohms.}$$

Thus the higher the wattage the lower is the resistance of the apparatus circuit and the greater the intensity of current that is used.

Apparatus using a current of more than 5 amperes must be connected to a power circuit or the intensity of current will exceed that which the fuse can transmit. Apparatus using a current of less than 5 amperes can be used on either type of circuit, but if the current is liable to approach 5 amperes it is unwise to connect it to a light point. Several light circuits are usually taken in parallel to each other from one fuse and the current that passes through the fuse is the sum of that in the individual circuits. Consequently the use of apparatus taking $4\frac{1}{2}$ amperes on one point would seriously limit the use of the others.

FUSES. A fuse is a weak point in a circuit which "blows" if a current of too great an intensity is passed. It consists of a short length of wire of a low melting point and if the current exceeds a certain intensity the heat generated melts the wire. This breaks the circuit, preventing further current flow and possible damage to another part of the wiring, or overheating which might cause a fire, also giving warning of the defect which caused the excess current. The fuse is placed in some situation where it is easily accessible and where the heat generated can cause no damage. It is an essential safety device in any wiring.

One type of fuse consists of a piece of suitable wire running through a tunnel in a porcelain holder. Each end of the wire is attached by a screw to a metal blade. The blades fit into metal sockets in a fixed porcelain base and the main wire is connected to the sockets (Fig. 82). The section containing the fuse wire can be removed for inspection and renewal of the wire. In another type of fuse, termed a cartridge fuse, the wire runs

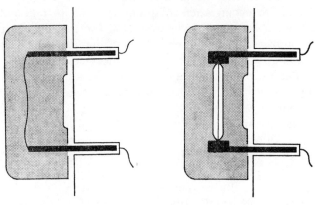

FIG. 82.—A FUSE.   FIG. 83.—A CARTRIDGE FUSE.

through a tube of glass or other suitable non-inflammable material which is held in position by metal clips and the whole tube is replaced when necessary (Fig. 83). In many cases there are fuses on both wires of the circuit, but if only one is provided it must be on the live wire. The use of one fuse, on the live wire only, has the advantage that if the fuse blows the live wire is always broken. If there is a fuse on each wire that on the neutral may blow, leaving the other intact, so that the apparatus circuit is still "live," with consequent danger of earth shock (Chapter 12).

In a physiotherapy department fuses should be included in the circuit of each piece of apparatus used for the treatment of patients, in addition to those in the department wiring. If a fault occurs, blowing of the apparatus fuse affects only one patient, whereas if one of the department fuses blows the current is cut off from all patients receiving treatment from this section of the wiring.

The blowing of a fuse is the result of the passage of a current of too great an intensity and this may arise in various ways. The current exceeds the permitted level if apparatus of too low a resistance, *i.e.* too high a wattage, is used, such as a 2,000 watt electric fire on a light circuit. If several parallel circuits are taken from one supply point the total current obtained is the sum of that in the individual circuits and may blow the fuse. This is liable to occur when adaptors are used to take extra circuits from a light or power point. A short circuit in the wiring or apparatus causes a reduction of the resistance and a current of large intensity passes. Such a short circuit may occur if the insulation round the flex connecting the apparatus to the source of supply becomes worn, so that the two supply wires come in contact with each other, or as a result of a connection between the live wire and earth.

If a fuse blows the apparatus which caused the damage should be disconnected and the main supply switched off. The faulty fuse is then identified, the ends of the old wire removed and a new wire of the correct thickness inserted, or, with the cartridge type, the whole tube is replaced. It is essential to use wire of the correct thickness. If it is too thick it is possible to pass a current of greater intensity than that which the rest of the wiring is designed to carry, with consequent risk of damage. If the wire is too thin the fuse blows at too low an intensity of current, causing considerable inconvenience.

POWER PLUGS. Apparatus working on a power circuit should be connected to the supply by a three point wall-plug. The pins to fit into the sockets are placed at the angles of a triangle, two being similar and the third either larger or differently spaced from the others, so that the plug can be inserted into the socket in one way only. The two similar pins are for connection of the apparatus circuit to the supply, and are marked "L" and "N" for the live and neutral wires. Some plugs incorporate a fuse on the live wire. This must not be capable of transmitting more than the 13 amperes that the main wiring is designed to carry, but should be selected according to the intensity of current used by the apparatus which it connects to the supply. In this way it safeguards both the main wiring and the apparatus circuit. Flex carrying three wires is used, and with the system of coding which has, up to the present, been employed in the United Kingdom the red wire is connected to the pin marked "L," the blue or black wire to that marked "N" and the green or brown wire to the third pin,

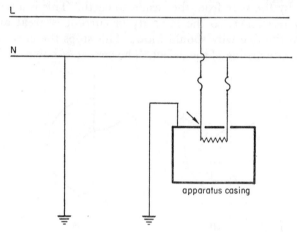

FIG. 84.—EARTHING OF APPARATUS CASING.

which is marked "E." In other countries different colourings have been used with a consequent risk of incorrect and dangerous connections. International agreement has now been reached, by which the live wire is coloured brown, the neutral blue and the earth green and yellow. Some time lapse must, however, be anticipated before this code is in universal use and in the meantime great care must be taken to ascertain the correct mode of connection. The wire connected to the pin marked "E" is for connection of the apparatus casing to earth. The socket into which it fits is earthed and the other end of the wire is connected to the apparatus casing. The third pin may operate a switch which disconnects the other two sockets from the source of supply when the plug is withdrawn, or a shutter which prevents contact with these sockets.

The earthing of the apparatus casing is a precaution against earth shock. If the apparatus casing is not earthed in this manner, and the insulation on the live wire becomes worn so that this wire comes in contact with the casing, any connection between the casing and earth completes a circuit through which current passes. If this connection is through some person he receives an earth shock. When the casing is correctly earthed, immediately the live wire comes in contact with it current passes by the wire from the casing to earth. This is a pathway of low resistance, so the intensity of current is great and the fuse on the live wire should blow. This stops the current flow and gives warning of the defect. The circuit is shown in Fig. 84,

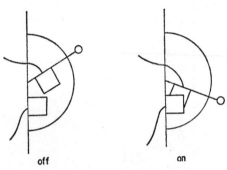

off   on

FIG. 85.—LIGHT OR POWER SWITCH.

the point at which the insulation is worn being indicated by the arrow. Exceptions to the need to earth apparatus casing occur when the casing is of non-conducting material and when the apparatus is "double insulated," making a connection between the live wire and the casing virtually impossible.

When connecting the wires to the screws inside the plug care should be taken that a minimal amount of insulation is removed from each, so that there is no danger of the exposed wires making contact with each other. The bridge which holds the wires in position as they enter the plug should be firmly secured, so that if any tension is placed on the flex, the danger of the wires being pulled away from their connections is reduced.

SWITCHES. The current is turned on and off by means of a

switch. Switches vary in type according to the intensity of current that is to be passed through them. The ones commonly used in houses and physiotherapy departments consist of two copper blades which fit into copper sockets (Fig. 85). When the switch is on, the blades are gripped in the sockets and the circuit completed. When the circuit is broken, a spring ensures the sudden separation of the sockets and blades. If they were parted slowly, arcing might occur, and the intense heat would gradually burn away the copper contacts. There is a switch for each light and power point and it is most satisfactory if this breaks both wires of the circuit. When this is not so it should be placed on the live wire, otherwise connection to the live wire can be made even when the switch is turned off and the danger of earth shock is increased (Chapter 12).

Other types of switch are encountered where very large or very small intensities of current are transmitted. Main switches and those operating such devices as electric cookers and immersion heaters carry a large intensity of current and so have

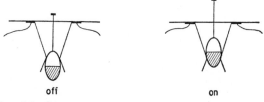

off   on

FIG. 86.—SWITCH FOR CURRENT OF SMALL INTENSITY.

long copper blades and a very strong spring. This is necessary in order that the break of the circuit shall be very sudden, as the danger of arcing is increased when the intensity of current is large. On the other hand, the switches of cell batteries used for the treatment of patients carry a very small intensity of current, and a simple push and pull type is used. The construction of this is shown in Fig. 86. Two sprung metal contacts are connected to the wires of the circuit. Between them is a rod on the end of which is a knob, the lower part of this being of metal, the upper part of some insulating material. When the rod is pulled up the metal part lies between the contacts and the circuit is made, when it is pressed down the insulation comes between the contacts, breaking the circuit. Closing the lid of the apparatus usually presses the rod down, so ensuring that the circuit is broken and wastage of the cells is avoided.

Cost of Electricity

The Board of Trade unit of electrical energy is the kilowatt hour, *i.e.* 1,000 watts for one hour, 100 watts for 10 hours, etc., and the number of units used is registered on the meter. The arrangement of the dials of the meter varies, but may be as shown in Fig. 87. In this case the first dial on the left records tens of thousands of units, the next one thousands and so on, the small dial below the others showing tenths of units, so a reading is taken straight across the dials. That in Fig. 87 is 20,915·1 units. Where the pointer is between two numbers, the lower one is read. Also marked on the meter are the voltage and type of current, information which may be of importance

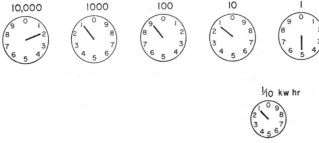

FIG. 87. READING OF ELECTRICITY METER.

to a physiotherapist when giving treatment in a patient's home, in order that she may know what apparatus can safely be used. There are different methods of charging for electric power. A fixed rate, based, for example, on the size of the house, may be charged, together with a small charge, *e.g.* twopence per unit. Alternatively there may be no basic rate but a higher charge for each unit used, usually between sixpence and ninepence. Sometimes a certain number of units are charged at the higher rate and any used beyond this at the lower one. If different rates are charged for light and power, the latter is the cheaper,

e.g. threepence to fourpence per unit, compared with eightpence
to ninepence for lighting. In this case the use of lighting equipment on the power circuits is not permitted. Electricity used
only during off-peak periods can be obtained at a lower cost
than the above, generally at about one penny per unit or less,
depending on the hours at which the supply is made available.

9

D.C. FOR THE TREATMENT
OF PATIENTS

DIRECT current for the treatment of patients may
be obtained from cells or from the A.C. main supply.
Although the constant D.C. is little used for this purpose
nowadays, the apparatus designed for its production may be
utilised to obtain the modified D.C.

The Cell Battery

A cell battery can conveniently be used to supply a direct
current for the treatment of patients. It has the advantages
that, being independent of the main supply, the dangers of
earth shock and of shock from failure of the main supply are
eliminated, also that the cells produce an absolutely constant
D.C. Its disadvantage is that the cells, which must be replaced
periodically, are expensive.

About 90 volts are required for the treatment of patients, so
60 dry Leclanché cells, connected in series, are used to supply
the circuit. These are in the form of a block battery, and are
connected through a switch to the coil of a potential divider,
which is usually of the circular type. The patient's circuit is
taken in parallel to this coil, and contains a moving coil
milliamperemeter in series with the patient's terminals. A
reversing switch may also be included in this circuit. The
circuit of the apparatus is shown in Fig. 88.

When the switch is turned on, current passes from the cells
through the switch and coil of the potential divider back to the
cells. The potential divider controls the intensity of current
supplied to the patient's circuit, as explained in Chapter 2.
In the patient's circuit the current passes through the milliamperemeter, reversing switch and patient's terminals. Care

must be taken to turn the switch off when the apparatus is not in use, as the current flows through the coil of the potential divider even when there is none in the patient's circuit, and the cells would be quickly used up.

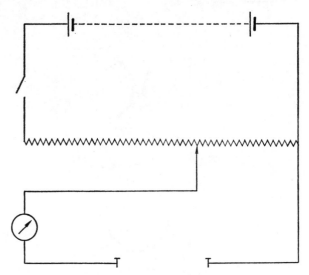

FIG. 88.—CIRCUIT OF CELL BATTERY FOR D.C.

THE REVERSING SWITCH (Fig. 89). This is a device for reversing the direction of the current supplied to the patient. There are various types of reversing switch, in one of which two semicircular metal strips are joined together with the convex surfaces towards each other, but separated by insulating material. Four equidistant contacts are arranged so that one touches each end of each strip. The contacts are fixed, but the strips can be rotated through a quarter of a circle by turning a knob. Two opposite contacts, A and B in Fig. 89, are connected to the source of current, and the other two opposite contacts, C and D, to the external circuit. In the upper diagram the course of the electron flow is to A, then to C and to the external circuit via X. The electrons return via Y to D, then to B, and so back to the source. In the lower diagram the strips have been rotated through a quarter of a circle. Again electrons flow to

A, but this time they pass to D, to the external circuit via Y, and return via X to C, pass to B, and so back to the source.

If a reversing switch is included in a circuit in which a one way reading milliamperemeter is used, the latter must be placed before the reversing switch.

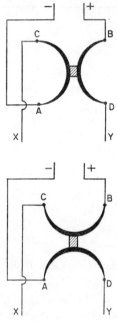

FIG. 89.—REVERSING SWITCH.

D.C. for the Treatment of Patients from the A.C. Main

The apparatus for obtaining, from the main supply, a D.C. for the treatment of patients may incorporate either metal rectifiers or a valve. The former is satisfactory for the low voltage required, but the latter may be used when the circuit forms part of a combined treatment unit in which valves are used for the production of other currents.

METAL RECTIFIER CIRCUIT (Fig. 90). The alternating main current is passed through a step-down static transformer which reduces the EMF to approximately 110 volts and makes

the current earth-free. Tappings on the primary coil of the
transformer enable the apparatus to be used on supplies of
different voltages. The secondary coil of the transformer is connected to a Westinghouse bridge circuit of metal rectifiers, the
number of which is sufficient for the 110 volts. There is some
loss of voltage in the rectifiers and an output of about 80 volts
is obtained. After passing through the rectifier the unidirectional pulsating current is smoothed by two condensers in shunt

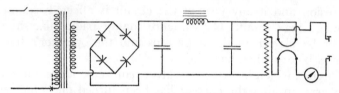

FIG. 90.—D.C. FROM A.C. MAIN, USING METAL RECTIFIERS.

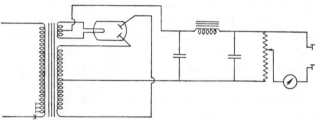

FIG. 91.—D.C. FROM A.C. MAIN, USING TWO-ANODE DIODE
VALVE.

and a choke coil in series with the output wires. The current
is then passed through a potential divider, from which the
patient's circuit is taken. This circuit consists of a milliamperemeter and the patient's terminals. A reversing switch may be
included. The working of all these components has been considered in preceding chapters.

VALVE CIRCUIT (Fig. 91). The metal rectifiers are
replaced by a diode valve with two anode plates. The current
from the secondary coil of the transformer is taken to the valve,
the circuit being arranged as in Fig. 75. The voltage is halved

by this arrangement and the pulsating D.C. obtained is smoothed and taken to a potential divider as before. The patient's circuit consists of a milliamperemeter and patient's terminals and possibly a reversing switch (not shown in Fig. 91).

Care of Apparatus

All apparatus should be kept clean and dry, dusted regularly and covered when not in use. Moisture is liable to cause corrosion and if any part of the circuit is affected extensive damage may result. Consequently damp pads, etc., should never be placed on the apparatus and the operator's hands should be dry when handling the equipment.

Circuits which incorporate valves require about one minute to warm up after the current has been turned on. Once the circuit has warmed up the current should be left on if the apparatus is required in a short time, as repeated heating and cooling shortens the life of the filament of a valve. Great care must be taken to leave the controls at zero and it is advisable to detach the leads from the patient's terminals while the apparatus is switched on but not in use, in order to eliminate the danger of electric shock from inadvertent contact with the electrodes.

The physiotherapist cannot repair defects in the circuits of modern electrical equipment, but should be able to remedy faulty wall plug and lead connections. If, when the apparatus is connected to the supply and switched on, the pilot lamp does not light, the wall plug connections may be at fault. If the pilot lamp lights but no current is obtained for the patient, the connection of the leads to the patient's terminals should be examined.

A cell battery requires renewal of the cells from time to time and this can be carried out by the physiotherapist. Inadequate output of current usually indicates that new cells are needed. The apparatus should be kept in a cool, dry place as dampness and warmth shorten the life of the cells.

10

PRODUCTION OF MODIFIED D.C.

Muscle Stimulating Currents

A CURRENT which varies in intensity can produce muscle contraction. A number of different types of current are used for muscle stimulation, and they can be divided into three groups:

(1) Currents providing stimuli of long duration, which may alternatively be classified as modified D.C. The impulses range from 10 to 2,000 milliseconds in duration and are infrequently repeated. Various wave forms are available, which are considered below.

(2) Currents providing stimuli of short duration, the impulses ranging from 0·01 to 1 millisecond in duration. Infrequently repeated stimuli are used for the testing of electrical reactions, but for treatment purposes they are commonly repeated 50 to 100 times per second and the current may then be classified as one of the faradic type.

(3) The sinusoidal current, which is a low frequency A.C., the graph being a sine curve and the frequency usually 50 cycles per second.

The production of the faradic and sinusoidal currents is considered in Chapter 11.

Modifications of the Direct Current

Interruption is the most usual modification of the direct current, the current flow commencing and ceasing at regular intervals. Occasionally the current is surged, so that the intensity increases gradually, then falls either suddenly or gradually. With the interrupted D.C. various types of impulse are available, depending on the following factors:

1. WAVE FORM. The intensity of the current may rise and fall suddenly so that the impulses are rectangular (Fig. 92 (1)), or the change may be gradual, as with the trapezoidal (Fig. 92 (2)), triangular (Fig.92 (3)) and saw-tooth (Fig. 92 (4)) impulses. In each case the important factor is the time required for the current to reach its maximum intensity, as this affects the response obtained when the current is used for the stimulation of nerve or muscle.

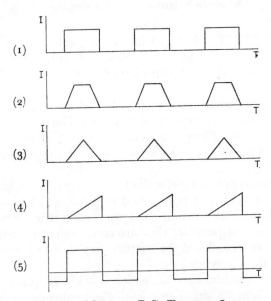

FIG. 92.—MODIFIED D.C. TYPES OF IMPULSE.
(1) Rectangular, (2) Trapezoidal, (3) Triangular,
(4) Saw–tooth, (5) Depolarised.

2. DEPOLARISATION. A current of low intensity may flow in the reverse direction during the interval between the impulses (Fig. 92 (5)). The current is no longer direct but its therapeutic effects are the same as those of the interrupted D.C. and the chemical formation which accompanies the passage of a D.C. through an electrolyte is reduced.

3. DURATION. Impulses with a duration of 100, 300 and 600 milliseconds are most commonly used for treatment with

the interrupted D.C. A greater range is required for the testing of electrical reactions, from 100 to 0·01 milliseconds, which includes stimuli of both long and short durations. In addition impulses of 1,000 and 2,000 milliseconds are available from some stimulators.

4. FREQUENCY. This is determined by the duration of the intervals between the impulses. The interval cannot usually be of shorter duration than the impulse, but its duration can be increased with consequent reduction of the frequency. Various frequencies are commonly available. That of 30 per minute is suitable for I.D.C. treatment with impulses which have a duration of 100 milliseconds, but if the duration of the impulse is increased the frequency should be reduced.

Production of Interrupted D.C.

The on and off switch can be employed for interrupting a current, but its use tends to weaken the spring and is not satis-factory for treatments. The method may be used if no other is available.

Various circuits incorporating valves or transistors may be used to produce an interrupted current. Their action is illus-trated by the multivibrator circuit shown in Fig. 95. The following description assumes the use of valves, and the principles underlying the working of the circuit are the switching action of the triode valve and the so-called C.R. timing circuits; certain points regarding the wiring of resistances in series are also relevant.

ACTION OF THE TRIODE VALVE. If a triode valve is connected into a circuit so that the anode is positive in relation to the filament, and the filament is heated, current passes across the valve. The grid lies between the filament and the anode. If it has no charge it has no effect on the current passing across the valve. If it is given a negative charge it reduces or, if the charge is strong enough, stops the flow of current across the valve, while if the grid has a positive charge it causes an increase in the intensity of current. As the grid lies closer to the filament than does the anode, a variation in the grid charge has more effect on the intensity of the current flowing across the valve than does a similar variation in the anode voltage. If a sufficiently strong negative charge is applied to the grid the current across the valve ceases, while if the grid loses this negative charge the current flows again. Thus the valve can act as a switch in the circuit.

C.R. Timing Circuits. When a condenser is connected to a source of supply it becomes charged. If it is then disconnected from the supply, and a circuit made between the plates, the condenser discharges through the circuit. This principle can be illustrated by the circuit shown in Fig. 93. When the switch is in position A the condenser is charged from

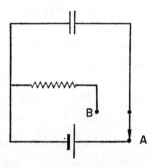

FIG. 93.—Circuit to Show Charge and Discharge of a Condenser.

the cell. When the switch is moved to position B the condenser discharges through the resistance. The time taken for the condenser to discharge depends on the capacity of the condenser and the resistance of the circuit (Chapter 6). The duration of the condenser discharge varies with $C \times R$

where C = capacity of the condenser measured in farads
R = resistance of the circuit measured in ohms.

Resistances in Series. When resistances are wired in series with each other the potential drop across each is directly proportional to its resistance. If two equal resistances (r_1 and r_2 in Fig. 94) are wired in series with each other and a P.D. of 100 volts is applied to the circuit, there is a P.D. of 50 volts across each resistance, as each is half the total resistance of the circuit. If r_1 is removed and replaced by a resistance which has one-third of the resistance of r_1, r_2 has three times the resistance of the new r_1, and forms three-quarters of the total resistance of the circuit. So the P.D. across r_2 rises to 75 volts, *i.e.* three-quarters of the total EMF, while that across

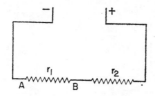

FIG. 94.—RESISTANCES IN SERIES.

the new r_1 is 25 volts. If r_1 is removed completely and a gap left in the circuit, no current flows. The resistance of the gap is infinite and compared with it the resistance of r_2 is negligible. The P.D. across the gap is the whole 100 volts and there is no P.D. across r_2. That is, the point A in the circuit is at the same potential as the negative supply line to which it is connected, while the point B is at the same potential as the positive supply line.

WIRING OF THE MULTIVIBRATOR CIRCUIT (Fig. 95). Two triode valves (V_1, V_2) are wired in parallel with each other across the supply lines. A resistance is placed between each anode and the positive supply line (Ra_1, Ra_2). In parallel with each valve are a condenser and a resistance, in series with each other (C_1R_1, C_2R_2). One plate of each condenser is connected to the anode of one valve (A_1, A_2), the other to the grid of the other valve (G_2, G_1).

WORKING OF THE MULTIVIBRATOR CIRCUIT. When the current is first switched on it passes equally across both valves, but a circuit of this type is very sensitive to interference from outside sources and almost immediately some electron disturbance causes a variation in the intensity of the current across one of the valves. The interference is similar to that which occurs in television reception. Rise or fall in the intensity of the current flowing through either valve initiates the action of the circuit, but if the change is a decrease in the intensity of

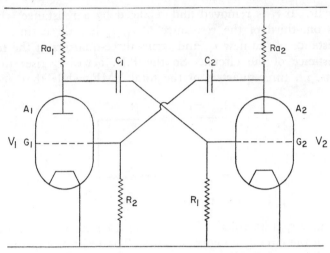

FIG. 95.—THE MULTIVIBRATOR CIRCUIT.

current across V_1 the following sequence of events takes place. In accordance with the principles of resistances in series, the potential drop between the supply lines is divided between V_1 and Ra_1 in direct proportion to their resistance. A decrease in the intensity of the current passing through V_1 corresponds to an increase in the resistance of the valve, and when this occurs the P.D. across it rises, and that across Ra_1 falls. The P.D. between A_1 and the positive supply line is reduced, and A_1 becomes more positive. The positive charge is transmitted through C_1 to the grid of the other valve (G_2) and causes an increase in the current across V_2. This corresponds to a fall in the resistance of V_2, so the P.D. across V_2 falls and that across Ra_2 rises. Thus the difference of potential between A_2 and the positive supply line is increased and A_2 becomes less positive, *i.e.* more negative. The negative charge is transmitted via C_2 to G_1, making it more negative and further reducing the intensity of the current across V_1. As before, this causes A_1 to become more positive and the charge is transmitted to G_2, resulting in a further increase in current across V_2. A_2 becomes less positive and the negative charge on G_1 is again increased. The process continues until G_1 is so negative that V_1 ceases to conduct. A_1 is then at the same potential as the positive supply line, so G_2 is more positive than at any other time and V_2 is transmitting maximum current. This is the switching action of the valves, and the series of events occurs instantaneously. The circuit is then stable, with one valve cut off and the other fully transmitting.

The condenser C_2 is in parallel to V_2 and so the P.D. across it is the same as that across the valve. It is charged at the beginning of the action, the left hand plate being negative and the right hand plate positive, but during the above sequence of events the P.D. across V_2 falls and so that across C_2 also falls. C_2 therefore begins to discharge through R_2 and V_2 and its left-hand plate gradually loses its negative charge. The grid of

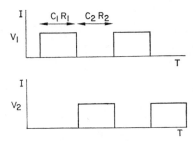

FIG. 96.—CURRENT THROUGH VALVES
OF MULTIVIBRATOR CIRCUIT.

V_1 is connected to this plate, with no resistance between, so is at the same potential as the condenser plate. Thus as the condenser discharges G_1 also loses its negative charge and when the charge falls to a certain level V_1 again begins to transmit current. The time that elapses before this occurs depends on the duration of the condenser discharge, which is determined by the product of the capacity of C_2 and the ohmic resistance of R_2. When V_1 begins to transmit current the switching action is again brought into play, but acting in the reverse direction to the previous occasion. Consequently V_2 is cut off and V_1 transmits maximum current. This state lasts until the discharge of C_1 through R_1 results in the reduction of the negative charge on G_2 and permits the passage of current through V_2, *i.e.* it is controlled by the product of C_1R_1.

F

Thus the current passes first through one valve, then through the other. The duration of the flow through V_2, during which V_1 is cut off, depends on C_2R_2. The duration of the flow through V_1, during which V_2 is cut off, depends on C_1R_1 (Fig. 96).

CURRENT SUPPLIED TO THE PATIENT. The patient's circuit is wired in parallel to Ra_2 and the interrupted current which flows through this resistance is also supplied to the patient. The periods of current flow occur when V_2 is trans-

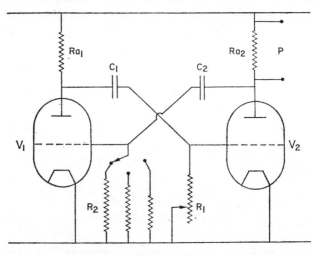

FIG. 97.—THE MULTIVIBRATOR CIRCUIT WITH VARIABLE RESISTANCES.

mitting and their duration is determined by C_2R_2. The intervals occur when V_2 is cut off and their duration is determined by C_1R_1. By using variable resistances for R_2 and R_1 the duration and frequency of the impulses can be adjusted. Increase in the resistance of R_2 increases the duration of the stimuli, while increase in the resistance of R_1 increases the intervals between them and so reduces their frequency. The circuit with variable resistances is shown in Fig. 97. The resistances may be varied either by using a series rheostat or by moving a switch so that a different resistance coil is included. In Fig. 97 the second of these methods is used for R_2, and three different pulse durations are available. R_1 is shown as a series rheostat and the intervals between the pulses are varied gradually. Either method can be used for each resistance, and may be observed in different apparatus. In some models definite pulse durations and frequencies are selected, in others either or both are varied gradually.

A circuit of this type can be modified to produce impulses with the various wave forms shown at the beginning of the chapter, and to provide depolarised impulses.

Production of Surged D.C.

The current can be surged by rotating the knob of a circular rheostat, but this tends to wear the wires of the rheostat, and should be used only when no other method is available. Surging is commonly carried out by an electronic device.

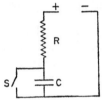

FIG. 98.—CIRCUIT TO ILLUSTRATE ELECTRONIC SURGER.

THE ELECTRONIC SURGER. Valves or transistors may be used in this device, the principles of which are illustrated by the circuit shown in Fig. 98. When the switch S is open the condenser C charges through the resistance R from the source of supply. As the circuit contains a resistance the charging is fairly slow. The P.D. between the condenser plates rises at first quickly, then more slowly, as the P.D. developed opposes the charging current. When the switch is closed a circuit of low resistance is completed between the plates. The condenser discharges rapidly through this circuit and the P.D. between its plates falls suddenly. The graph in Fig. 101 (2) shows the P.D. across the condenser.

In the surger circuit (Fig. 99) a triode valve may be used to replace the switch. It is connected to a source of interrupted

D.C. in such a way that the grid receives a negative charge during the periods of current flow. The interrupted D.C. supplied from a multivibrator circuit may be used for this purpose. When the grid of the triode valve has a negative charge the valve will not conduct current and the condenser

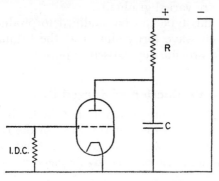

FIG. 99.—ELECTRONIC SURGER CIRCUIT.

charges from the source of D.C. The charge is fairly slow and the P.D. between the plates rises at first quickly, then more slowly, as in the preceding example. When the grid loses its negative charge the valve becomes capable of conducting a

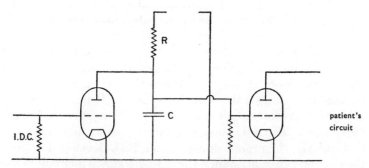

FIG. 100.—ELECTRONIC SURGER CIRCUIT.

current and the condenser discharges across the valve. This is a circuit of low resistance and the discharge is rapid, so the P.D. between the condenser plates falls quickly. Thus the condenser charges during each period of flow of the interrupted

D.C. and discharges when the current ceases (Fig. 101 (1) and (2)).

Another triode valve is included in the circuit in which the current to be surged is flowing, and from which current is supplied to the patient (Fig. 100). The condenser is connected to this in such a way that the grid becomes positive when the condenser is charged, so causing an increase in the intensity of

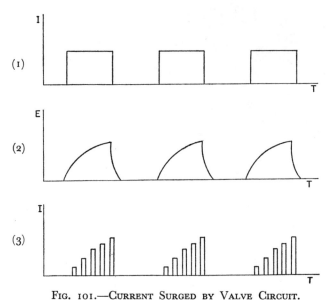

FIG. 101.—CURRENT SURGED BY VALVE CIRCUIT.
(1) Interrupted D.C. supplied to grid of triode valve,
(2) P.D. across condenser, (3) Surged current.

current in this circuit. When the condenser discharges the grid loses its positive charge and the intensity of current falls again. Thus the current varies in intensity as the P.D. across the condenser varies, rising gradually in intensity, then falling suddenly, and the graph of a surged D.C. would be the same as that of the P.D. across the condenser (Fig. 101 (2)). This is the type of surge produced by most electronic apparatus.

The duration of each surge is the same as the duration of the flow of the interrupted D.C. supplied to the first valve, the intervals between the surges equal the intervals of the interrupted D.C. Thus if the interrupted D.C. is supplied from a multivibrator circuit the duration and the frequency of the surges are controlled by the resistances in this circuit.

The same device can be used to surge other types of current. This is considered further in Chapter 11, but Fig. 101 (3) shows the graph of a surged current of the faradic type.

11

FARADIC AND SINUSOIDAL APPARATUS

The Faradic Current

THE term faradism was originally used to signify the type of current produced by a faradic coil, which is a type of induction coil. The current provided by the first faradic coils was an unevenly alternating current, each cycle consisting of two unequal phases, the first of low intensity and long duration, the second of high intensity and short duration. The frequency was approximately 50 cycles per second and the duration of the second phase, which was the effective one, about 1 millisecond. The graph of this current is shown in Fig. 102. A number

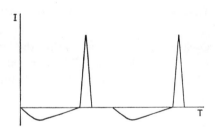

FIG. 102.—THE ORIGINAL FARADIC CURRENT.

of different types of faradic coil were developed, but the only one of these now in use is the Smart-Bristow faradic coil. The current it produces differs from that described above in that a train of damped oscillations, with a frequency of about 1,000 cycles per second, follows each peak of high EMF (Fig. 103). The peaks of EMF and first few oscillations of each group are the effective stimuli. Faradic coils have now been largely superseded by electronic stimulators. These supply currents which produce the same physiological effects as the original faradic current, although often differing considerably from them in wave form. The features essential for the production

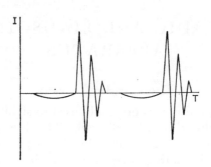

FIG. 103.—FARADIC CURRENT FROM SMART-BRISTOW COIL.

of these physiological effects are that impulses with a duration of between 0·1 and 1 millisecond are repeated 50–100 times per second. One such current is shown in Fig. 104.

Faradic Current from an Electronic Stimulator

Various types of electronic stimulator are available, and although the so-called faradic currents that they produce differ somewhat in wave form, they all fulfil the essential conditions that impulses with a duration of 0·1 to 1 millisecond are repeated 50 to 100 times per second.

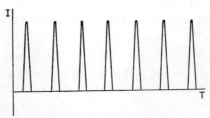

FIG. 104.—FARADIC TYPE OF CURRENT FROM ELECTRONIC STIMULATOR.

PRODUCTION. A current of the faradic type can be produced by the multivibrator circuit described in Chapter 10.

Referring to Fig. 95, page 128, R_2 controls the duration of the impulses, and in order that they shall have the short duration typical of the faradic current, this resistance is reduced to a suitably low value. R_1 controls the length of the intervals between the impulses, and therefore their frequency, so this also must have a low resistance to provide the necessary high repetition rate. The current may be depolarised by a reverse wave between the impulses, in order to reduce chemical action, although if the duration of the impulses is very short this is unnecessary, as the chemical formation is negligible.

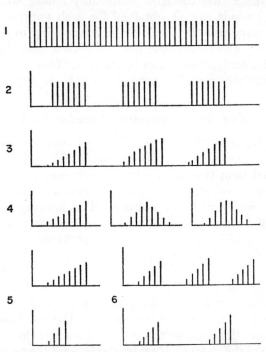

FIG. 105.—FORMS OF THE FARADIC CURRENT AVAILABLE FROM MODERN STIMULATORS (EACH STROKE REPRESENTS ONE IMPULSE).
(1) Unmodified, (2) Interrupted, (3) Surged, which may vary in (4) Wave Form, (5) Duration, (6) Frequency of Surges.

MODIFICATION (Fig. 105). The faradic current is commonly modified, usually by surging, occasionally by interrupting. In most modern stimulators an electronic device is used to surge the current. The action of this is described in Chapter 10 and the circuit can be modified to give surges of various durations, frequencies and wave forms. In a combined treatment unit the surger circuit is often controlled by that producing modified D.C., and in this case the duration and frequency of the surges are regulated by the controls that regulate the duration and frequency of the long duration impulses. It is desirable that the durations of the surges and intervals between them should be regulated by separate controls, in order that the most satisfactory muscle contractions and rest periods can be obtained for each patient. Various forms of surge may be available, corresponding to the trapezoidal, triangular and saw-tooth impulses, and that most suitable for each patient must be selected. These various types of surge are shown in Fig. 105.

The Smart-Bristow Faradic Coil

THE CIRCUIT (Fig. 106). The apparatus comprises two circuits, the primary and the secondary. The primary circuit is supplied from two dry Leclanché cells wired in series, and consists of a switch, interrupting device and primary coil, wired in series with each other. The interrupting device consists of a metal screw, held in a screw support, and with a lock nut by which it can be fixed in position. This prevents it from being shaken out of position by the continual vibration of the hammer against it. The tip of the screw rests against the sprung metal limb of a hammer, which is arranged so that it vibrates in a horizontal plane, as this facilitates an even action and interruption of the current. The soft iron head of the hammer lies opposite to the core of a small electromagnet. The limb of the hammer is prolonged beyond the head, and on this part of it is an adjustable weight, which enables the speed of vibration to be altered. The tip of the screw and the point on the limb of the hammer with which it makes contact are faced with platinum or tungsten. These hard metals resist the wear which tends to occur from the sparking and from the continual vibration of the hammer against the screw. Between the screw support and the base of the hammer is wired a condenser. The primary coil is wound on a hollow wooden bobbin.

The secondary coil is wound over the primary coil and contains more turns of wire. The ends of the secondary coil are usually connected to a potential divider, from which the patient's circuit is supplied. A laminated soft iron core can be inserted into the hollow wooden bobbin on which the primary

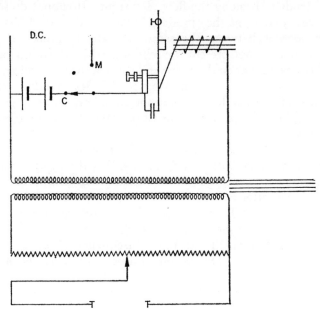

FIG. 106.—THE SMART-BRISTOW FARADIC COIL.

and secondary coils are wound. The end of this bobbin lies opposite to the hole in the side of the case of the apparatus.

WORKING. When the switch is turned on current passes from the cells through the switch, screw support, screw, limb of the hammer, electromagnet and primary coil back to the cells. As the current passes through the electromagnet coil a magnetic field is set up, the core of the coil is magnetised and attracts the soft iron head of the hammer. This draws the limb of the hammer away from the screw and the circuit is broken.

The current ceases, the electromagnet loses its magnetic field, the head of the hammer is released and the limb of the hammer springs back against the screw, making the circuit again. This series of events is repeated 50 to 100 times per second and an interrupted D.C. flows in the primary circuit. This circuit has inductance, so as the current varies a self-induced EMF is set up, which opposes the rise of the primary current, making it more gradual. When the primary current falls the self-induced EMF tends to prolong the flow of current. It cannot do so to any great extent, as the circuit is broken, and instead charges the condenser between the screw and the hammer. If the condenser were not present the self-induced EMF would cause sparks to pass between the screw and the hammer, so prolonging the flow of current and making its fall less sudden. The presence of the condenser does not completely eliminate the sparking, but it does much to assist the rapid fall of the current intensity.

The condenser then discharges back round the primary circuit, the reverse flow of current assisting the rapid collapse of the magnetic fields around the primary coil and the electromagnet, the latter ensuring the immediate release of the head of the hammer. The circuit is of low ohmic resistance, with inductance, and so the condenser discharge produces a train of damped oscillations. These have a frequency of about 1,000 cycles per second. The graph of this current is shown in Fig. 107 P.

The varying current flowing in the primary coil sets up a varying magnetic field which cuts the secondary coil, producing an EMF in it by electromagnetic induction. Lenz's law states that the induced EMF is in the opposite direction to the force producing it, and Faraday's law of electromagnetic induction that the strength of the induced EMF is proportional to the rate of change of the magnetic field. Therefore, when the primary current is rising in intensity the induced EMF is in the opposite direction to that applied to the primary and, as the rise of current is slow, is of low voltage (Fig. 107A). When the primary current falls the induced EMF is in the same direction as that applied to the primary and, because the fall is rapid, is of high voltage and short duration (Fig. 107B). It is followed by a train of damped oscillations (Fig. 107c). Because the variations in the primary current are so rapid, they tend to produce a high EMF in the secondary coil, and it is not

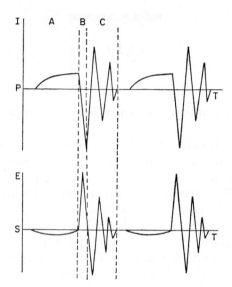

FIG. 107.—CURRENT FROM SMART-BRISTOW FARADIC COIL.

necessary to have a secondary with very many more turns of wire than the primary in order to produce an adequate voltage. The maximum output from the secondary circuit is about 40 volts.

FUNCTIONS OF THE CONDENSER. The primary function of the condenser is to reduce the sensory stimulation that is produced by the current. It does this by assisting the rapid fall of the primary current, in the manner described above. The peak of EMF induced in the secondary coil is consequently of short duration and high voltage, and the secondary coil need not have very many more turns of wire then the primary. This, together with the short duration of the impulses, ensures a minimum of sensory stimulation. In addition the condenser reduces the sparking between the screw and the hammer, and so the wear on the contact points.

REGULATION OF CURRENT. When the iron core is inserted into the bobbin on which the primary and secondary coils are wound, it concentrates the magnetic field and increases

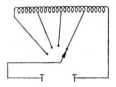

FIG. 108.—LAYER STUD REGULATING DEVICE.

the EMF that is induced in the secondary circuit. The current is surged by inserting and withdrawing the iron core. Most modern coils have a potential divider for regulation of the current. When this is used the required intensity can be selected and the core inserted fully at each surge. In some of the older models a layer stud regulating device replaces the potential divider. A secondary circuit with this method of regulation is shown in Fig. 108. The secondary coil is wound in four layers and a selector switch enables one, two, three or all of these layers to be connected to the patient's terminals. Thus $\frac{1}{4}$, $\frac{1}{2}$, $\frac{3}{4}$ or all of the secondary coil may be used, a corresponding proportion of the voltage being available for the patient. This provides four different current strengths, and fine regulation is obtained by inserting the core for the necessary amount at each surge.

Care of Faradic Coils

The care of apparatus considered in Chapter 9 applies where appropriate to the faradic coil, but certain additional points require attention.

If the hammer fails to vibrate when the current is switched on, the defect is in the primary circuit. The interrupting device may be at fault and its operation can often be initiated by tapping the hammer gently towards the electromagnet. This is the direction in which the hammer normally moves, and forcing in the other direction may strain the sprung limb. The screw may require adjustment, and when this is so the lock nut is loosened, the screw adjusted until the hammer vibrates and the locknut tightened again. Failure to obtain current in the primary circuit may be due to worn or dirty contacts between the screw and the hammer, or to a broken connection. Alternatively the cells may need renewal.

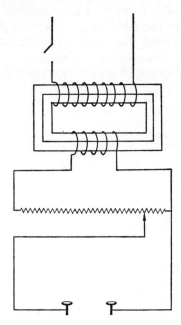

FIG. 109.—CIRCUIT FOR OBTAINING SINUSOIDAL CURRENT.

If the hammer vibrates but no current passes to the patient, the defect is in the secondary circuit. There may be a faulty connection of a lead to a terminal, or a broken wire in some part of the circuit.

The cover of the coil should be closed when it is not in use, but nothing should be placed inside the lid, or the hammer may be forced out of its correct alignment.

The Sinusoidal Current

The sinusoidal current is an evenly alternating, low frequency current. The graph (Fig. 13, page 21) is a sine curve and the frequency is usually 50 cycles per second. This is the type of current produced by an A.C. dynamo and supplied from the A.C. main.

SINUSOIDAL CURRENT FROM THE A.C. MAIN (Fig. 109). About 60 volts are required for the treatment of patients with the sinusoidal current. A step-down transformer is employed to lower the EMF of the main supply and to make the current earth-free. The intensity of the current from the secondary of the transformer is regulated by a potential divider, and it is surged by an electronic surger (not shown in Fig. 109.)

12

ELECTRIC SHOCK

A SHOCK is a painful stimulation of sensory nerves which is caused by a sudden flow, cessation or variation in the intensity of a current passing through the body. Motor nerves may also be stimulated, causing a muscle contraction.

THE SEVERITY OF THE SHOCK. The greater the intensity of the current which passes through the body, the more severe is the shock. In accordance with Ohm's law, the current intensity depends on the EMF and the resistance. A high EMF is liable to produce a current of large intensity, and so the EMF available for the patient is limited to the maximum likely to be required for the treatment. It is recommended that apparatus for constant D.C. should make available not more than 75 volts, that for muscle stimulating currents 110–130 volts, depending on the type of current. A high resistance reduces the intensity of current. If exposed parts of the circuit are touched with damp hands the shock is more likely to be severe than if the hands are dry, while severe shocks may be experienced in baths, because the resistance of the skin is lowered by soaking in water.

The severity of the shock also depends on the path taken by the current and a strong current through the head, neck, heart or whole body might prove fatal. Shocks are generally more severe with the alternating than with the direct current, because the intensity of the former is continually changing and so it provides stronger sensory stimulation; also it may produce tetanic muscular contractions, which make it impossible for the victim to let go of the conductor.

EFFECTS OF SHOCK. Following a minor shock the victim may be frightened and distressed, but does not lose consciousness. After more severe shock there is a fall in blood pressure and possibly loss of consciousness. In extreme cases, there is cessation of respiration, which may be accompanied by cardiac arrest, due to ventricular fibrillation resulting from electrical stimulation of the heart. Cessation of respiration is recognised by lack of respiratory movements and cyanosis; cardiac arrest by absence or abnormality of respiratory movements, absence of pulse in the *carotid* artery and fully dilated pupils.

TREATMENT OF SHOCK. In the event of a shock occurring the first step is to disconnect the victim from the source of supply. A.C. should be switched off at once but unvarying D.C. reduced slowly if possible, as sudden cessation of current causes a second shock. If there is no switch in the circuit the victim must be removed from contact with the conductor, but the rescuer must take care not to receive a shock himself in doing so. Contact with the affected person should be made only through a thick layer of insulating material.

Following a minor shock the patient is reassured, and allowed to rest. Water may be given to drink, but hot drinks should be avoided as they cause vasodilatation and sweating, and consequently further fall in blood pressure. In all cases it is advisable to consult a medical officer. If the shock is more severe the victim is laid flat in such a position that respiratory passages are clear, tight clothing is loosened and plenty of air allowed. Undue warmth is avoided as it causes vasodilatation, sweating and a fall in blood pressure; also because external heat increases metabolism and so the demand for oxygen, of which there is already a dearth in the tissues. If the patient is unconscious nothing is given by mouth and a medical officer is summoned without delay. If respiration has ceased the airway is cleared and artificial respiration commenced immediately by the mouth to mouth or mouth to nose method, or oxygen administered by a bag and mask. In the event of cardiac arrest external cardiac massage must be applied in addition to the above and in both cases it is essential to call immediately for medical help. All persons liable to be called upon to deal with such an emergency should receive instruction in artificial respiration and external cardiac massage, with practice on a dummy.

Causes of Shock and Precautions

A patient may receive a shock in the course of an electrical treatment as a result of a sudden increase in the intensity of the current. This may occur if a direct or low frequency current is switched on with the controls turned up or if insufficient time is allowed for the apparatus to warm up, so that the current comes on suddenly after the controls have been turned up. It can also occur if the intensity control is turned up unduly during the intervals in the flow of an interrupted or surged current, if there is some fault in the apparatus, most often in the potentiometer, or if the patient touches an exposed part of the circuit. With the constant D.C. sudden cessation of current also causes a shock but this does not occur with A.C. or modified D.C. as the current is continually rising and falling in intensity.

To avoid the occurrence of shocks in these ways, all apparatus should be tested before use and connections checked. Controls should be checked to ensure that they are at zero before switching on, adequate warming up time allowed and the current intensity increased with care. Patients should never be allowed to touch electrical equipment and all apparatus should be serviced regularly by a competent electrician.

The physiotherapist may receive a shock when handling equipment, if two live parts of the circuit are touched at the same time. Apparatus should always be disconnected from the source of supply before faults are investigated.

When light contact is made between two conductors which are charged to different electrical potentials a spark passes between them. Such sparking may occur on touching short-wave diathermy electrodes to which current is applied, or on making contact with the metal casing of apparatus, especially the edges and corners where charges concentrate. Sparking causes unpleasant sensory stimulation but is not dangerous and should not really be classed as an electric shock.

A shock may be the result of a connection to earth, and this is considered below.

Earth Shock

When a shock is due to a connection between the live wire of the main and earth it is known as an earth shock.

THE EARTH CIRCUIT. Electric power is transmitted by one live cable and one neutral cable which is connected to earth (Chapter 5). The earth forms part of the conducting pathway and any connection between the live wire of the main and earth completes a circuit through which current passes. If some person forms part of this circuit he receives an earth shock (Fig. 110, Circuit A). Thus an earth shock is liable to

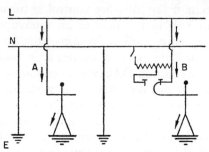

FIG. 110.—SIMPLE CIRCUIT FOR EARTH SHOCK.

occur if any person makes contact with the live wire of the main while connected to earth.

CONNECTION TO THE LIVE CABLE. A patient who is receiving treatment with a current that is not earth-free is connected to the live cable. Such a connection can also be made by touching an exposed part of the circuit, and if the switch breaks only the neutral wire the connection can be made even when the switch is turned off (Fig. 110, Circuit B). If the insulation on the live wire is faulty and the wire comes in contact with some metal part of the apparatus, such as the casing or the reflector of an infra-red lamp, this part of the apparatus provides a connection to the live cable.

CONNECTION TO EARTH. This may be made by touching any conductor which is connected to earth, such as gas or water pipes, radiators or stone floors, particularly if they are damp. A metal bed on such a floor, or which is in contact with a pipe or radiator, forms an earth connection, also the casing of apparatus if it is, correctly, connected to earth.

EXAMPLES OF EARTH SHOCK. Simultaneous connection to the live wire and to earth can occur in a variety of ways, for instance if a patient who is receiving treatment with a current that is not earth-free rests her hand on a water pipe, or if a physiotherapist, while holding an electrode that is connected to the live wire, touches the earthed apparatus casing. Also if some person who is standing on a damp stone floor touches the casing of apparatus which is not connected to earth and with which the live wire is in contact.

PRECAUTIONS AGAINST EARTH SHOCK. Physiotherapy departments should be arranged so that there is minimal danger of making an earth connection while in contact with apparatus. Water and gas pipes should be out of reach of the apparatus and of patients receiving treatment. The floor should be of insulating material and should be kept dry, as water seeping through cracks in linoleum to a stone floor beneath can form an earth connection. If the floor is not of insulating material a rubber mat should be placed under the patient's feet during electrical treatments.

Switches must break the live wire and fuses must be on the live wire, so that if an earth circuit is made and a large current passes the fuse blows and stops the current flow. The metal casing of all apparatus must be connected to earth (Chapter 8).

Patients should not be permitted to touch the apparatus during treatment and especial care must be taken when currents are administered in baths, as in these circumstances an earth connection is easily made. The bath must be of insulating material and leaking baths must not be used, as a trickle of water may form a connection to earth. The bath should have no fixed taps or waste pipe and if a rubber hose is used for filling the bath it must be removed before treatment is begun, as when it is damp a current can pass along it. Water should not be added to the bath during the treatment.

Currents used for the treatment of patients should always be earth-free and most types of modern electromedical apparatus supply an earth-free current. The current obtained from cells is always earth-free and that from the A.C. main can be rendered so by a static transformer, but to ensure safety it is important that the construction of the transformer is in accordance with the specified regulations and it is advisable to ascertain that this is so when purchasing equipment.

13

ELECTRICAL STIMULATION OF NERVE AND MUSCLE

Stimulation of a Nerve

A NERVE impulse can be initiated by an electrical stimulus. To achieve this a varying current of adequate intensity must be applied.

A NERVE IMPULSE. When a nerve fibre is in its resting state there is a difference of potential between the outer and inner surfaces of the plasma membrane. The outer surface bears a positive charge, the inner surface a negative charge. In this state the plasma membrane is not permeable to sodium ions, these positive ions accumulate on its outer surface, and there is an associated arrangement of other ions, following a definite pattern, inside and outside the membrane. If the P.D. across the membrane falls below a certain level, the membrane

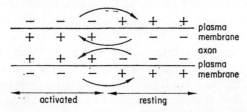

FIG. 111.—TRANSMISSION OF A NERVE IMPULSE.

becomes permeable to sodium ions. A nerve impulse is initiated if any factor causes the P.D. across the plasma membrane of the nerve cell or fibre to fall below this level. When this occurs the sodium ions begin to enter the axon, causing a further fall in the P.D. and increase in the permeability of the membrane to the ions. There is also a re-arrangement of the other ions, and the process builds up until there is a reversal of the P.D., the outer surface of the membrane becoming negative, the inner one positive. Currents are now set up between this activated part of the nerve and the adjacent area, which is still in its resting state (Fig. 111). The currents result in restoration of the resting P.D. in the activated part of the nerve fibre and a fall in that across the plasma membrane of the adjacent area. The sequence of events described above then takes place in this area. Thus the reversal of P.D. is transmitted along the nerve, and is an essential feature of a nerve impulse.

ELECTRICAL STIMULATION. If an electric current of sufficient intensity is applied to the body, a nerve impulse can be initiated. The plasma membrane of the nerve fibre forms a resistance, which lies in series with the other tissues, so a P.D.

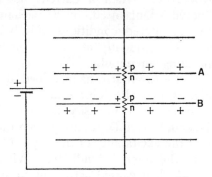

FIG. 112.—ELECTRICAL STIMULATION OF A NERVE FIBRE.

is set up across it as the current flows. The surface of the membrane nearer to the cathode becomes negative in relation to the opposite surface. In Fig. 112 the surfaces of the plasma membranes marked "n" lie nearest to the cathode and so become more negative, while the surfaces marked "p," lying nearer to the anode, become more positive. On the side of the nerve nearer to the anode (A in Fig. 112) this increases the resting P.D. across the membrane, but on the side of the nerve nearer to the cathode (B in Fig. 112) the additional charges are of the opposite polarity to those present on the resting membrane, and so reduce the P.D. across it. If the P.D. falls below the level at which the membrane becomes permeable to sodium ions, these ions begin to enter the axon and the series of events described above takes place. Thus a nerve impulse is initiated.

An impulse is initiated if the P.D. falls sufficiently across any part of the plasma membrane of the nerve cell or fibre. If the cathode is applied over a superficial nerve, the side of the nerve nearest to the electrode (B in Fig. 112) is activated, but if the anode is applied it also can cause the initiation of a nerve impulse. In this case it is the aspect of the nerve further from the electrode (B in Fig. 112) that is activated. The current spreads in the tissues, so the current density is rather less on the further surface of the nerve fibre than on the nearer one, and in consequence the anode is less effective than the cathode in initiating an impulse.

ACCOMMODATION. When a current flows at constant intensity the nerve adapts itself, by a mechanism not fully understood, to the altered conditions, this being known as accommodation. Consequently an unvarying current is not effective in initiating an impulse. When the current rises in intensity the impulse is initiated as described above, but a fall in current intensity can also initiate an impulse. While the current flows at constant intensity accommodation of the nerve takes place and the P.D. resulting from the current flow no longer affects the excitability of the nerve fibre, which has adapted itself to the altered conditions. When the current ceases the P.D. which it caused across the plasma membrane suddenly disappears, so altering the total P.D. across the membrane. On the aspect of the nerve nearer to the anode (A in Fig. 112) the extra P.D. was augmenting that across the resting membrane, and its sudden loss causes a fall in the P.D. If this fall is to the level at which the membrane becomes permeable to sodium ions, an impulse is initiated. A fall in the intensity of current is less effective than a rise in initiating an impulse. It is the side of the nerve nearer to the anode that is affected, and so the anode produces a greater stimulation than the cathode.

Because the nerve has the property of accommodation a current which rises or falls suddenly in intensity is more effective in initiating an impulse than one which changes slowly. If the variation of current is gradual there is time for accommodation to take place, and a greater intensity is needed to be effective, than if the variation is sudden. A current that changes very slowly does not initiate a nerve impulse.

EFFECT OF THE NERVE IMPULSE. When a nerve impulse is initiated at a nerve cell or end organ, there is only one direction in which it can travel along the axon, but if it is initiated at some point on the nerve fibre it is transmitted in both directions from the point of stimulation.

When a sensory nerve is stimulated the downward travelling impulse has no effect, but the upward travelling impulse is appreciated when it reaches conscious levels of the brain. If impulses of different durations are applied, using the same intensity of current for each, it is found that the sensory stimulation experienced varies with the duration of the impulse. The impulses of long duration produce an uncomfortable, stabbing sensation, but this becomes less as the duration of the impulses is reduced until, with impulses of 1 millisecond and less, only a mild, prickling sensation is experienced.

When a motor nerve is stimulated, the upward travelling impulse is unable to pass the first synapse, as it is travelling in the wrong direction, but the downward travelling impulse passes to the muscles supplied by the nerve, causing them to contract.

Stimulation of Innervated Muscle

When a stimulus is applied to a motor nerve trunk, impulses pass to all the muscles that the nerve supplies below the point at which it is stimulated, causing them to contract. When the current is applied directly over an innervated muscle the nerve fibres in the muscle are stimulated in the same way. The maximum response is obtained from stimulation at the motor point, which is over the point at which the main nerve enters the muscle or, in the case of deeply placed muscles, at the point where the muscle emerges from under cover of the more superficial ones.

TYPE OF CONTRACTION. When a single stimulus is applied, impulses pass simultaneously to a number of motor units so that, in normal circumstances, there is a sudden brisk contraction, followed by immediate relaxation. If a succession of stimuli are applied at infrequent intervals, *e.g.* one stimulus per second, each produces an isolated muscle contraction, and there is time for complete relaxation between the impulses. Increase in the frequency of the stimuli shortens the periods of relaxation and, when the frequency exceeds 20 per second, there is not time for complete relaxation between the contractions, so partial tetany results. Further increase in the frequency reduces the amount of relaxation until, when the frequency exceeds 60 per second, there is no perceptible relaxation and the contraction is fully tetanic.

STRENGTH OF CONTRACTION. This depends on the number of motor units activated, which depends on the intensity of the current applied, and on certain other factors, which are considered below.

RATE OF CHANGE OF CURRENT. A current which changes suddenly in intensity is found to be more effective in producing a contraction of innervated muscle than one which changes gradually. This is because the latter allows time for accommodation of the nerves. If the intensity of current rises suddenly, as with the rectangular impulses (Fig. 92 (1), page 124), there is no time for accommodation to take place and a muscle contraction results. If the current rises more slowly, as with the trapezoidal, triangular and saw-tooth impulses (Fig. 92), there is some accommodation and a greater intensity of current is needed to produce a contraction than with the sudden rise. The slower the rate of change of the current, the greater is the intensity needed to be effective, and a current which rises and falls very slowly does not produce a muscle contraction.

DURATION OF STIMULUS. To demonstrate the effects of stimuli of different durations an interrupted D.C. with rectangular impulses is used and impulses with durations of 0·01, 0·03, 0·1, 0·3, 1, 3, 10, 30 and 100 milliseconds should be available. The current is applied to a normally innervated muscle, using first the impulse with a duration of 100 milliseconds, and increased until a minimal contraction is obtained.

The intensity of current is noted, then the impulse shortened and the intensity of current needed to produce a contraction again observed. This procedure is repeated for each duration of stimulus in turn. It is found that the stimuli of longer durations, *i.e.* down to a variable point, usually between 10 and 1 or between 1 and 0·1 millisecond, produce a muscle contraction with the same intensity of current for all durations of stimulus, but when the impulse is shortened beyond this point, a greater intensity of current is required each time the duration of the impulse is reduced. With the impulses of shorter durations, the briefer the period for which the current flows, the greater is the intensity needed to cause the P.D. across the plasma membrane of the nerve to fall to the critical level at which a nerve impulse is initiated. With the impulses of longer durations the time for which the current flows does not affect the response obtained. This is because there is time for accommodation of the nerves, which takes place before the flow of current is completed, so that only the first part of each stimulus is effective.

A graph can be plotted of the intensity of current against the duration of the stimulus, or the effective voltage may be recorded instead of the intensity of current. Such a graph is termed a strength-duration curve. A logarithmic scale is used, as this magnifies the part of the curve showing the effects of the stimuli of shorter durations, which would otherwise be difficult to observe. The curve shown in Fig. 113 is typical of normally innervated muscle.

The chronaxie and rheobase can be read from the strength-duration curve. The rheobase is the minimum intensity of current that will produce a response if the stimulus is of infinite duration, in practice an impulse of 100 milliseconds being adequate for assessing this. The chronaxie is the minimum duration of impulse that will produce a response with a current of double the rheobase. So if the rheobase is 6 milliamperes, the chronaxie is the duration of the shortest impulse that will produce a muscle contraction with a current of 12 milliamperes. The chronaxie of normally innervated muscle is short, often being less than 1 millisecond.

POLE USED FOR STIMULATING. A nerve impulse can be

initiated by either a rise or a fall in the intensity of current, but the former is the more effective and is commonly used for nerve stimulation. When the current rises in intensity the cathode is more effective than the anode in initiating a nerve impulse, so, provided that the intensity of the current is not altered, the contraction obtained when the cathode is placed over the nerve or muscle is stronger than that obtained when

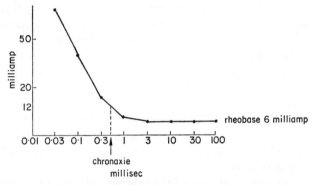

FIG. 113.—STRENGTH–DURATION CURVE OF NORMALLY INNERVATED MUSCLE.

the anode is used. This can be demonstrated by applying the anode and cathode at some distance from each other, interrupting the current at infrequent intervals and observing the relative strengths of the resulting muscle contractions.

Stimulation of Denervated Muscle

When a current is applied to denervated muscle, the muscle fibres can be stimulated directly. The manner in which this is brought about is similar to that in which a nerve fibre is stimulated, there being changes in the potential difference across the plasma membrane of the muscle fibre. Denervated muscle does not react to the electrical stimuli of shorter durations so readily as does the motor nerve, but provided that the intensity of the current and duration of the stimulus are adequate, contraction of the muscle results. As each muscle fibre must be stimulated directly, the maximum response occurs when the current passes through the greatest number of fibres, so is usually obtained with a longitudinal application, one electrode being placed over each end of the muscle belly.

TYPE OF CONTRACTION. A single stimulus causes an isolated muscle contraction, but this and the relaxation are less sudden than when the muscle is stimulated through its motor nerve, and is described as "sluggish." To demonstrate the contraction it is advisable to use impulses with a duration of at least 100 milliseconds, and these cannot be repeated with sufficient frequency to produce tetany.

STRENGTH OF CONTRACTION. This depends on the number of muscle fibres stimulated, therefore on the intensity of the current, and on certain other factors which are considered below.

RATE OF CHANGE OF CURRENT. The property of accommodation is much less marked in denervated muscle than in nerve. Consequently a current that does not rise immediately to maximum intensity is as effective in producing a contraction as one that rises suddenly. An impulse that rises slowly in intensity, such as the trapezoidal, triangular and saw-tooth impulses, can produce a contraction of denervated muscle with an intensity of current which is less than that required to produce a contraction of innervated muscle. For this reason such impulses are termed selective.

DURATION OF STIMULUS. To observe the effects of stimuli of different durations, the current is applied to a muscle whose motor nerve has degenerated, the procedure being the same as that described for innervated muscle. The strength-duration curve can be plotted, and is found to be different in shape from that obtained when the motor nerve is intact (Fig. 114). The intensity of current has to be increased each time the duration of the impulse is reduced. This occurs because denervated muscle has not the same property of accommodation as has the motor nerve. The whole of each stimulus is effective, so the longer the duration, the less is the intensity of current needed to cause the necessary fall in the P.D. across the plasma membrane of the muscle fibre. Muscle contractions are not obtained with the impulses of very short durations and, although the point at which the response is lost is variable, the curve rises steeply to infinity.

The rheobase may be less than that of innervated muscle, but the chronaxie is longer, often being more than 1 millisecond.

POLE USED FOR STIMULATING. When stimulating denervated muscle it is often found that the contraction pro-

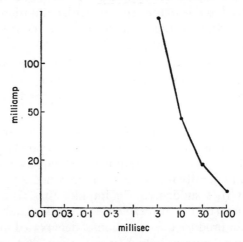

FIG. 114.—STRENGTH-DURATION CURVE OF DENERVATED MUSCLE.

duced when the anode is the stimulating electrode is stronger than that obtained with the same intensity of current when the cathode is used. This does not always occur and the reason for it is not known, but when the anode produces a better response than the cathode it is used as the active electrode for treatment purposes.

14

THE FARADIC AND SINUSOIDAL
CURRENTS

The Body as a Conductor of Electricity

THE tissues of the body are capable of transmitting an electric current because the tissue fluids contain ions and so are electrolytes. Consequently the current which passes through the body is a convection current, consisting of a two-way migration of ions, and the conductivity of the different tissues varies according to the amount of fluid that they contain. Muscle, for example, has a good blood supply and so is a good conductor, while fat is a poor conductor. The current tends to travel in those tissues which have a low resistance, although it is not always possible for it to avoid the high resistance layers. The epidermis has a high resistance, 1,000 ohms or more, as it contains little fluid and the superficial layers do not readily absorb moisture. The current must pass through the epidermis and appropriate measures are used to reduce its resistance when applying electrical treatments. Passage of a convection current may result in chemical changes, which can constitute a danger in some treatments.

Physiological Effects of the Faradic Type of Current

The name "faradism" was originally applied to the current obtained from a faradic coil. This was an unevenly alternating current, each cycle consisting of two unequal phases, the first of long duration and low EMF, the second of short duration and high EMF (Fig. 102, page 135). The duration of the second phase was about 1 millisecond, and the frequency 50 cycles per second. Modern apparatus has made available various types of current which, while differing considerably in wave form, produce the same physiological effects as the original faradic current. These may be classed as currents of the faradic type. The essential features are that stimuli with a duration of 0·1–1 millisecond are repeated 50–100 times per second.

STIMULATION OF SENSORY NERVES. When a current of the faradic type is applied to the body, a mild prickling sensation is experienced. This is due to stimulation of the sensory nerves, and is not very marked, because the stimuli are of fairly short duration. The sensory stimulation causes a reflex vasodilatation of the superficial blood vessels, so that there is slight reddening of the skin, or erythema. The vasodilatation is probably confined to the superficial tissues, and is of little practical value.

STIMULATION OF MOTOR NERVES. A current of the faradic type stimulates the motor nerves, and so, provided that the current is of sufficient intensity, causes contraction of the muscles which they supply. Because the stimuli are repeated 50 times per second or more, the contraction is tetanic. If this type of contraction is maintained for more than a short period of time, muscle fatigue is produced, so the current is commonly surged or interrupted to allow for muscle relaxation. When the current is surged the contraction gradually increases and decreases in strength, in a manner similar to a voluntary contraction. When the current is interrupted the contraction commences and ceases suddenly, being maintained during the period of current flow.

EFFECTS OF MUSCLE CONTRACTION. When a muscle contracts as a result of electrical stimulation, the changes taking place within the muscle are similar to those associated with voluntary contraction. There is increased metabolism, with a consequent increase in the demands for oxygen and foodstuffs, and an increased output of waste products, including metabolites. The metabolites cause dilatation of capillaries and arterioles, and there is a considerable increase in the blood supply to the muscle.

As the muscles contract and relax they exert a pumping action on the veins and lymphatic vessels lying within and around them. The valves in these vessels ensure that the fluid they contain is moved towards the heart. If the muscle contractions are sufficiently strong to cause joint movement this also exerts a pumping effect. Thus there is increased venous and lymphatic return.

If a muscle contracts a sufficient number of times against the resistance of an adequate load there is increase in bulk of the fibres and the muscle is strengthened. There is some doubt whether the muscle contractions caused by faradic stimulation can produce these effects, but presumably if sufficient contractions are produced against the resistance of an adequate load it should be possible for them to do so.

EFFECTS ON DENERVATED MUSCLE. The intensity of current required to produce a contraction of denervated muscle with an impulse lasting for 1 millisecond is usually too great to be tolerable for treatment purposes. Therefore the faradic type of current is not satisfactory for the stimulation of denervated muscles.

POLE USED FOR STIMULATING. With the faradic coils no polarity is marked on the terminals because the current is alternating, but a muscle contraction should be produced most easily if the active electrode is connected to the terminal that is negative during the high peak of current. On some types of electronic apparatus the polarity of the terminals is marked, and this refers to the polarity during the high peak of current, which is the effective stimulus. The active electrode should be connected to the cathode, as this produces a contraction of innervated muscle with less current than is required at the anode.

CHEMICAL EFFECTS. When a D.C. is passed through an electrolyte chemical changes take place at the electrodes. If the chemicals formed come in contact with the tissues there is a danger of electrolytic burns, although the danger is appreciably less with an intermittent than with a constant D.C. When the current is alternating the ions move one way during one phase of current, in the reverse direction during the other phase, and if the two phases are equal the chemicals formed during one phase are neutralised during the next phase. If, however, the reverse wave of current is not equal to the

G

forward wave, there are some chemical changes, which could cause an electrolytic burn, but this danger is not so great as with a direct current. The current obtained from a faradic coil flows equally in both directions and there is no chemical formation. That obtained from electronic apparatus may have a greater flow in one direction than the other, but if the impulses are of very short duration the chemical formation should not be great enough to give rise to a serious danger of burns. It is, however, advisable to take appropriate precautions.

Physiological Effects of the Sinusoidal Current

The sinusoidal current is an evenly alternating low frequency current. The frequency is usually 50 cycles per second, which provides 100 stimuli per second, each lasting for 10 milliseconds.

STIMULATION OF SENSORY NERVES. When the sinusoidal current is applied to the body a marked prickling sensation is experienced. This is due to the stimulation of the sensory nerves, and is more marked than that produced by the faradic type of current, as the stimuli are of longer duration. Because of this marked stimulation of the superficial sensory nerve endings there is appreciable reflex vasodilatation. A definite erythema of the skin is produced, and it is assumed that there is an increased flow of blood through the underlying tissues.

STIMULATION OF MOTOR NERVES. The sinusoidal current stimulates the motor nerves and, provided it is of sufficient intensity, causes contraction of the muscles which they supply. Because the stimuli have a frequency of 100 per second the contraction is tetanic, so the current is usually surged, occasionally interrupted, to allow for muscle relaxation. Owing to the marked sensory stimulation the current is not so comfortable as those of the faradic type. When applied locally it is not always possible to tolerate a great enough intensity to produce a muscle contraction.

EFFECTS OF MUSCLE CONTRACTION. These are the same as the effects of the muscle contractions produced by the faradic current, *i.e.* increased metabolism, improved blood supply to the working muscles, increased venous and lymphatic return and possibly strengthening and increase in bulk of the muscles.

EFFECTS ON DENERVATED MUSCLE. It is often possible to obtain a contraction of denervated muscle with a stimulus of 10 milliseconds, but the intensity required with the sinusoidal current would be too uncomfortable for treatments, so it is not used for producing contractions of denervated muscles.

CHEMICAL EFFECTS AND POLE USED FOR STIMU-LATING. As the current is an evenly alternating one, no chemical actions take place and there is no danger of chemical burns. Both phases of each cycle are identical, and so the active electrode may be connected to either terminal.

Therapeutic Effects and Uses of Faradic and Sinusoidal Currents

The faradic and sinusoidal currents are used primarily to produce contractions of normally innervated muscles, the current usually being surged so that the contraction gradually increases and decreases in strength. The resulting contraction has the closest resemblance to a voluntary contraction of any that can be produced by electrical stimulation.

The physiological effects of the two currents are similar, and so they could be used for the same purposes, but the sinusoidal current is little used nowadays. The small amount of sensory stimulation experienced with faradism makes it much more suitable than the sinusoidal current for localised muscle stimulation, although the latter can satisfactorily be applied in baths, and if a generalised effect is required may be preferred to faradism.

FACILITATION OF MUSCLE CONTRACTION. When a patient is unable to produce a muscle contraction, or finds difficulty in doing so, electrical stimulation may be of use in assisting voluntary contraction. This is evident when contraction is inhibited by pain or recent injury and it is probable that the electrical stimulation facilitates voluntary contraction through the muscle spindle mechanism.

When a voluntary contraction is performed impulses pass from the small anterior horn cells (A in Fig. 115) to the intrafusal muscle fibres, causing them to contract. The resulting tension activates the receptor organs in the muscle spindles (Fig. 115 M.S.) and impulses pass from them to the spinal cord. These increase the excitability of the large anterior horn cells (B in Fig. 115) and so facilitate the transmission of impulses to the extrafusal muscle fibres of the motor units (Fig. 115 M.U.),

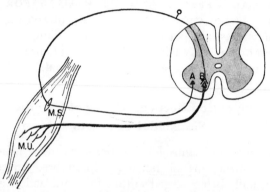

FIG. 115.—MUSCLE SPINDLE CIRCUIT.

which then contract. At the same time the impulses from the muscle spindles cause inhibition of the antagonists of the contracting muscles. Pain has an inhibitory effect on the large anterior horn cells, so impeding the transmission of impulses to the motor units. If the afferent nerve fibres from the muscle spindles are stimulated electrically, this should reduce the inhibition, so facilitating the transmission of voluntary impulses to the muscle, and also inducing relaxation of its antagonists.

When muscle contraction is inhibited by pain or recent injury, as, for instance, when active contraction of the quadriceps is impossible in painful rheumatoid arthritis of the knee joint or after menisectomy, faradic stimulation may be of assistance in establishing voluntary contraction. The treatment must be arranged so that the part is in a pain-free position and no movement causing pain is produced, as this would inhibit the discharge from the large anterior horn cells. Voluntary contraction should be attempted at the same time as the faradic stimulation and assistance from the latter is required only until a good voluntary contraction can be performed unaided.

RE-EDUCATION OF MUSCLE ACTION. Inability to contract a muscle voluntarily may be the result of prolonged disuse or incorrect use, as is seen, for example, in the intrinsic foot muscles in a longstanding flat foot, or the abductor hallucis in hallux valgus. In these circumstances faradic stimulation may be used to produce contractions, and so help to restore the sense of movement. The brain appreciates movements, not muscle actions, so the current should be applied in such a way that it causes the movement that the patient is unable to perform. Active contractions should be attempted at the same time as the electrical stimulation, the treatment being a preliminary to active exercise. It will probably take longer to establish a voluntary contraction than in those cases where inhibition is due to pain or injury, but once a satisfactory contraction can be performed electrical stimulation should be discontinued.

TRAINING OF A NEW MUSCLE ACTION. After tendon transplantation, or other reconstruction operations, a muscle may be required to perform a different action from that which it previously carried out. A new movement pattern has to be established. The muscle is stimulated with the faradic current, so that its new action is performed, and the patient must concentrate on the movement and attempt to assist with voluntary contractions. In this way the new muscle action may be taught, although it will take longer to achieve this than to re-educate an action which the muscle has previously performed.

EXERCISE FOR PARALYSED MUSCLES. In cases where there is neurapraxia of a motor nerve, impulses from the brain are unable to pass the site of the lesion to reach the muscles supplied by the affected nerve. Consequently voluntary power is reduced or lost. There is, however, no degeneration of the nerve, so that if it is stimulated with faradism below the site of the lesion, impulses pass to the muscles, causing them to contract. Electrical stimulation is not usually necessary in neurapraxia as recovery takes place without any marked changes in the muscle tissue, but, provided that there is no degeneration of the motor nerve, faradism may be used to exercise the paralysed muscles until the nerve begins to conduct impulses again. The faradic stimulation, combined with attempted active movement, helps to restore normal function, but is of use only until such time as a good voluntary contraction is established.

When a nerve has been severed, degeneration of the axons takes place and there is no longer a satisfactory response to faradism. This process takes several days to become complete, and for a few days after the injury a muscle contraction may be obtained with the faradic current. If this is so, faradism may be used to exercise the muscle so long as a good response is present, but must be replaced by modified D.C. as soon as the response begins to weaken.

There is little indication for the use of faradism in the treatment of incomplete nerve lesions. If a faradic response is present, it is largely the innervated muscle fibres that contract, and even if these are not already capable of active contraction, an early return of voluntary power can be expected. In a recovering nerve lesion voluntary power usually returns before the response to faradism, so any fibres responding to this current would be those capable of active contraction, while there would be little or no response of those whose nerve supply had not yet been restored.

STRENGTHENING AND INCREASED BULK OF MUSCLE. In order to increase the bulk and power of a muscle it is necessary for it to contract an adequate number of times against the resistance of a suitable load, and these conditions must be fulfilled if a muscle is to be strengthened as a result of electrical stimulation. When a muscle is very weak the weight of the part of the body that it moves forms an adequate load and under these circumstances electrical stimulation can be of assistance in restoring muscle bulk and power. The method may be used when for some reason, such as inflammation of or injury to the joint concerned, adequate active exercise is not possible. The electrical stimulation is an accessory to such active exercise as can be performed, and when adequate active exercise is possible the latter is a more satisfactory method of restoring muscle power than electrical stimulation. It is better for the patient that the results of the treatment should depend on his own efforts; active exercise is of more value than electrical stimulation in restoring normal function, and unless the muscle is very weak it is not practicable to provide an adequate load during electrical stimulation.

INCREASE IN BLOOD SUPPLY. Increased blood supply is brought about primarily by the vasodilatation in the working muscles, but also to some extent by the reflex effect of the sensory stimulation. Consequently the treatment is most effective if many muscles are made to contract and if a large area of skin is stimulated. For these reasons the current is usually applied in baths when used for this purpose, and the sinusoidal may be preferred to the faradic current, on account of the greater sensory stimulation that it produces. The treatment may be used for circulatory defects, such as chilblains, or following a long period of immobilisation. It is sometimes used in lower motor neurone lesions, such as anterior poliomyelitis, but the effect is reduced if muscle contractions are not obtained.

Occasionally the sensory stimulation alone is relied upon to increase the blood supply, in which case the sinusoidal current is preferable to faradism. The current is applied in a bath and is not surged, the intensity being kept below that required to produce a muscle contraction. This method may be used for improving the blood supply to areas where loss of cutaneous sensation renders heat treatments unsafe.

IMPROVED VENOUS AND LYMPHATIC DRAINAGE. Increased venous and lymphatic return is brought about by the pumping action of the alternate muscle contraction and relaxation, and of joint movement, on the veins and lymphatics. The treatment is most effective if the current is applied by the method described as faradism or sinusoidal under pressure (page 181), and may be used in the treatment of œdema, and sometimes for gravitational ulcers.

Faradic or sinusoidal baths can be used for mild cases of

œdema, but have the disadvantage that the limb must be dependent, and so gravity opposes the venous and lymphatic return.

PREVENTION AND LOOSENING OF ADHESIONS. When there is effusion into the tissues adhesions are liable to form, but these can be prevented by keeping the structures moving on each other. If adequate active exercise is not possible, electrical stimulation may be used for this purpose. Adhesions which have formed may be stretched and loosened by muscle contractions, *e.g.* muscles or tendons bound down by scar tissue. When a generalised effect is required sinusoidal baths are satisfactory, but for localised application the faradic current is more comfortable.

Technique with Faradic and Sinusoidal Current Treatments

Various methods of applying the faradic and sinusoidal currents can be used, according to the effects required. The technique of application of the faradic current for stimulation of individual motor points is described in detail, and can be adapted for the other methods mentioned.

PREPARATION OF APPARATUS. Either the Smart-Bristow faradic coil or an electronic stimulator may be chosen, the latter probably having an automatic surger. The operator tests the apparatus by attaching leads and electrodes to the terminals, holding the two electrodes in a moistened hand, inserting the core if a Smart-Bristow coil is being used, and turning up the current until a mild prickling sensation is experienced and a muscle contraction produced. If the surging is automatic the duration and frequency of the surge should also be tested.

The active electrode may be a disc electrode, or a small lint pad with a flat plate electrode. The latter is preferable for large muscles like the quadriceps and glutei, as it is easier to mould to the surface, so obtaining good contact. A flat plate electrode and lint pad are used for the indifferent electrode, to complete the circuit. The pads consist of at least eight layers of lint, so that they are thick enough to make good contact with the tissues and with the electrode and to absorb any chemicals which might be formed. They should be folded evenly with no creases, or there will be uneven distribution of current and consequent discomfort. The pads and lint covering the disc electrode are soaked in warm 1 per cent. saline. Tap water can be used but the addition of salt reduces the resistance of the solution, 1 per cent. saline having a rather lower resistance than the tissue fluids. Electrodes should be half an inch smaller all round than the pads, to reduce the danger of their coming in contact with the skin and causing uncomfortable concentration of current and possible damage to the tissues from chemical actions. Corners of electrodes should be rounded as points may become bent and dig into the pad, again causing concentration of current.

PREPARATION OF THE PATIENT. Clothing is removed from the area to be treated and the patient supported comfortably in a good light. It is important that she is warm, otherwise the muscles do not respond well to the stimulation. It is usually easiest to obtain muscle contractions in response to electrical stimulation if the part is supported so that the muscles are in a shortened position. It may, however, be desirable to modify this position according to the effects required. If the aim of treatment is to re-educate a muscle action, the patient may be arranged so that movement is produced when the muscle contracts, e.g. for training the quadriceps, the knee may be arranged in slight flexion so that extension takes place when the muscles are stimulated. In some cases movement can be obtained by supporting the limb in slings during the treatment, e.g. when training the deltoid muscle, movements of the shoulder joint can often be produced if the arm is supported in slings, though rarely from any other position. The joint movement should, however, be avoided if it causes pain, with consequent inhibition of muscle action.

APPLICATION OF ELECTRODES. The skin has a high resistance to an electric current as the superficial layers, being dry, contain few ions. The resistance is reduced by washing with soap and water to remove the natural oils and moistening with saline immediately before the pads are applied, in order to provide ions. Breaks in the skin cause a marked reduction in resistance which would result in concentration of the current and discomfort to the patient, so are protected by a little petroleum jelly[1] covered with a small piece of non-absorbent cotton wool to protect the pad. The indifferent electrode is applied to a suitable area, and when selecting this area the main consideration is that the electrode shall not cause contractions of muscles other than those being treated, and particularly not of their antagonists. Over the nerve trunk supplying the group of muscles to be treated is frequently a suitable position, *e.g.* above the medial epicondyle of the humerus for the flexor muscles of the forearm. Care must be taken not to cover the motor points of any of the muscles to be stimulated. For instance, when treating the anterior tibial muscles and peronei the indifferent electrode may be placed on the lateral aspect of the knee, but if it is too low it may cover the motor point of peroneus longus. In some cases it is not convenient to place the indifferent electrode over the nerve trunk supplying the muscles, and then any suitable area may be chosen; *e.g.* for the muscles of the shoulder girdle it may be placed on the upper part of the anterior chest wall. The indifferent pad should be large, to reduce the current density under it to a minimum. This prevents excessive skin stimulation and also, if it is not possible to avoid covering the motor points of some muscles, reduces the likelihood of unwanted muscle contractions. The indifferent electrode may be bandaged or fixed with a rubber strap, or body weight may be sufficient to hold it in position. If the pad is bandaged in position, or if it is liable to come in contact with the patient's clothing, it is covered with jaconet, rather larger than the pad, to protect the bandage or clothing from moisture.

APPLICATION OF CURRENT. The active electrode is placed over the motor point of the muscle to be stimulated. The motor point is the point at which the best contraction is obtained, usually being situated over the point at which the main nerve enters the muscle. This is frequently at the junction

[1] The most familiar form of petroleum jelly is Vaseline, made by the Chesebrough Manufacturing Co. Ltd.

of the upper and middle one-thirds of the fleshy belly of the muscle, although there are exceptions, *e.g.* the motor point of vastus medialis, whose nerve enters the lower part of the muscle, is situated a short distance above the knee joint. Deeply placed muscles may be stimulated most satisfactorily where they emerge from beneath the more superficial ones, *e.g.* extensor hallucis longus in the lower one-third of the lower leg. The exact position of the motor points varies in different individuals. Approximate positions of some motor points are shown in Figs. 116–121, but the most satisfactory method of determining their position is to consider the anatomy of the muscle to be stimulated.

The active electrode must be held firmly in position, a small pad in the palm of the hand, a disc electrode between the index and middle fingers. Firm contact ensures a minimum of discomfort and where possible the whole of the operator's hand should be in contact with the patient's tissues, so that she can feel the strength of the contractions produced.

The intensity of current is gradually increased until a good

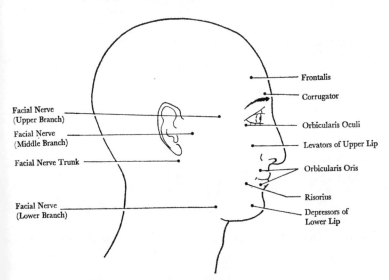

FIG. 116.—MOTOR POINTS OF MUSCLES SUPPLIED BY THE FACIAL NERVE.

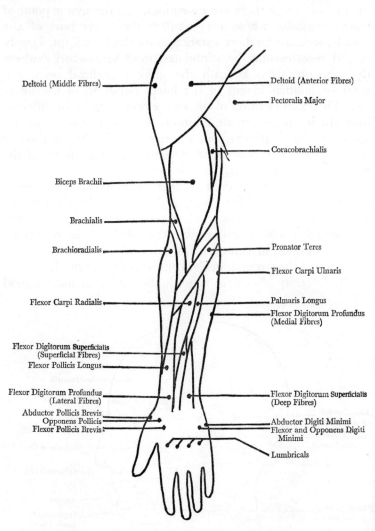

FIG. 117.—MOTOR POINTS OF THE ANTERIOR ASPECT OF THE RIGHT ARM.

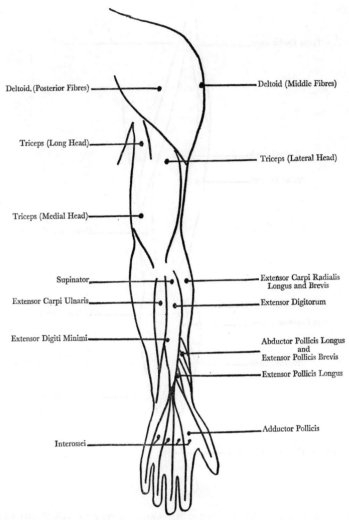

Deltoid. (Posterior Fibres)

Deltoid (Middle Fibres)

Triceps (Long Head)

Triceps (Lateral Head)

Triceps (Medial Head)

Supinator

Extensor Carpi Radialis
Longus and Brevis

Extensor Carpi Ulnaris

Extensor Digitorum

Extensor Digiti Minimi

Abductor Pollicis Longus
and
Extensor Pollicis Brevis

Extensor Pollicis Longus

Adductor Pollicis

Interossei

FIG. 118.—MOTOR POINTS OF THE POSTERIOR ASPECT OF THE RIGHT ARM.

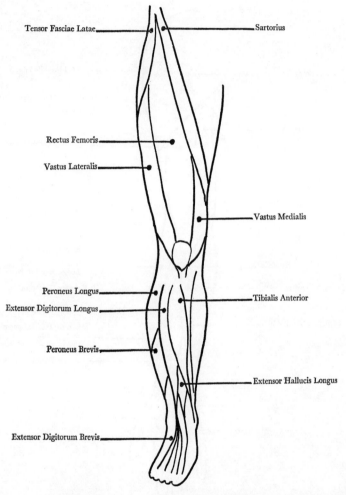

FIG. 119.—MOTOR POINTS OF THE ANTERIOR ASPECT OF THE RIGHT LEG.

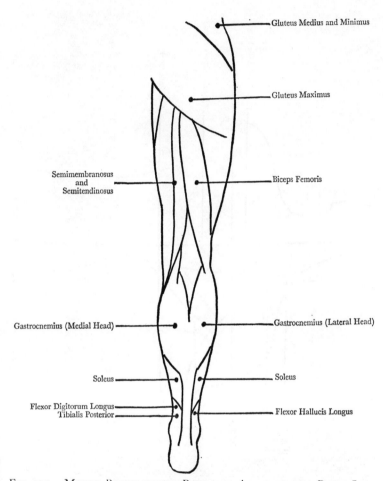

FIG. 120.—MOTOR POINTS OF THE POSTERIOR ASPECT OF THE RIGHT LEG.

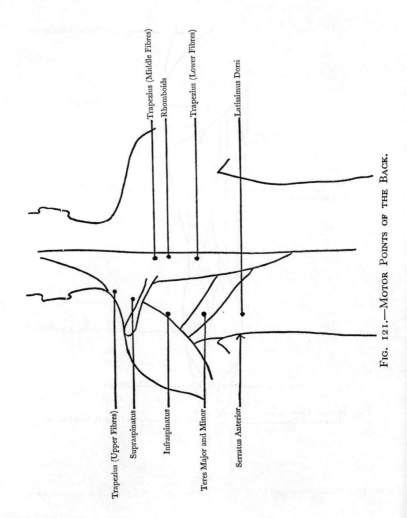

Trapezius (Middle Fibres)
Rhomboids
Trapezius (Lower Fibres)
Latissimus Dorsi

Trapezius (Upper Fibres)
Supraspinatus
Infraspinatus
Teres Major and Minor
Serratus Anterior

FIG. 121.—MOTOR POINTS OF THE BACK.

muscle contraction is obtained at the maximum point of each surge, then the surging continued to produce alternate contraction and relaxation of the muscle. When using the Smart-Bristow coil the current is surged manually by inserting and withdrawing the iron core. The surging must be rhythmical, and can be performed most satisfactorily if the operator's forearm is supported, movement taking place at the wrist joint. The speed of surging varies for different muscles, but should be such that a good contraction, followed by complete relaxation, is obtained. The surging should not be too slow, or the treatment is uncomfortable. Manual surging has the advantage that the strength and duration of each muscle contraction are easily controlled by the operator. When an automatic surger is used care must be taken that a suitable duration and frequency of surge are selected. This method has the advantage that the operator has one hand free, so that if necessary she can palpate tendons, etc., to ensure that the required action is being produced. Voluntary contractions may be attempted at the same time as those produced by the electrical stimulation, particularly when the current is being used to re-educate muscle action, and active exercises may be interspersed with the electrical treatment.

The duration of the treatment depends on the condition of the patient's muscles and on the purpose for which it is being used. When, for instance, electrical stimulation is used to re-educate muscle action the duration of the treatment session is determined by the length of time for which the patient can concentrate on the movement and assist in its production. When the aim is to strengthen the muscles each treatment should be continued so long as satisfactory muscle contractions are obtained, in order to ensure that each muscle performs as many contractions as possible. Muscle fatigue is indicated by weakening of the contraction, but does not occur rapidly with faradic stimulation. Treatments lasting 20–30 minutes can satisfactorily be given and 90 contractions of each muscle is generally regarded as the minimum treatment that can be effective. Usually 20–30 contractions are produced on one motor point, then the electrode is moved to another muscle. When all the muscles have been stimulated the operator returns to the first one, and the procedure is repeated. This sequence is continued for the duration of the treatment.

Methods of Application

STIMULATION OF MOTOR POINTS. This method, which is described in the preceding section, has the advantages that each muscle performs its own individual action, and that the optimum contraction of each muscle can be obtained. It has the disadvantage that, if there are many muscles to be stimulated, it is impossible to produce a large number of contractions of each.

STIMULATION OF MUSCLE GROUPS. With this method all the muscles of a group work together. Two fixed electrodes are used, one placed either over the nerve trunk supplying the group of muscles, or over their origin; the other so that it covers the motor points, or over the lower ends of the fleshy bellies of the muscles. All the muscles of the group work together, and so it is a satisfactory method for re-educating the action of muscles which normally work as a group, such as the quadriceps or small muscles of the foot. The method also permits many more contractions to be elicited from each muscle than if individual motor points are stimulated. In addition it may be used for large muscles with a multiple nerve supply, such as the abdominal or longitudinal back muscles. Great care must, however, be taken that a satisfactory contraction of each muscle in the group is obtained. If some muscles contract less strongly than others, because they are weaker or more deeply placed, the method is not suitable.

LABILE TREATMENT. An indifferent electrode is applied, as for the stimulation of motor points, and the second electrode moved over the area to be treated. The active electrode may be either a disc or a small pad with a plate electrode. The current is not surged, but as the electrode approaches and leaves the motor point of a muscle, that muscle contracts and relaxes. It is more difficult to gauge the required intensity of current than when the electrode is applied directly to the motor points, and the sensory stimulation is more marked. The method may, however, be used for treating large muscles with a multiple nerve supply, such as the longitudinal back muscles.

NERVE CONDUCTION. If a motor nerve trunk is stimulated, contractions are produced of all the muscles that it supplies beyond the point of stimulation. For this method of stimulation an indifferent electrode is applied to a convenient area, and the active electrode to some point at which the nerve trunk is superficial. It is not always desirable to produce simultaneous contractions of all the muscles supplied by one nerve, but on some occasions this is the most satisfactory method of application. The motor points may be inaccessible, owing to a wound or splinting, or if the limb is œdematous the current spreads in the fluid, and so it may be difficult to obtain contractions on attempting to stimulate the motor points. It is the most comfortable method of stimulating the muscles of facial expression. For this purpose three points over the branches of the facial nerve are stimulated, one behind the lateral corner of the eye, one in front of the ear, and one just above the angle of the jaw (Fig. 116).

BATH TREATMENTS. Both the faradic and sinusoidal currents may be applied in baths, the current usually being surged and of adequate intensity to produce muscle contractions. The sinusoidal current is sometimes used unsurged and at a low enough intensity to avoid muscle contraction. Application of the current in baths has the advantages that the water makes perfect contact with the tissues, the encumbrance of pads and electrodes is avoided and the prolonged soaking reduces the resistance of the skin. Widespread effects are produced and the method is particularly useful when the principal aim of treatment is to improve the blood supply to the area. The main disadvantages are that the treatment cannot easily be localised and that although many muscles are stimulated they do not all contract to the same degree, those which are strongest and most superficial responding most readily. Also the limb must be dependent, so gravity opposes the drainage of fluid from the part. The danger of electric shock is greater than with other methods, as earth connections are easily made. Also, soaking in water reduces the skin resistance, so that a small variation in the EMF causes a considerable variation in the intensity of current. For this reason the controls should be turned up very slowly. It is unnecessary to wash the part before treatment, but breaks in the skin must be protected with petroleum jelly and metal objects removed from the area, in order to avoid concentration of current. The water in the baths should be comfortably warm but the temperature not unduly high as soaking in hot water may prove exhausting for the patient.

The baths may be arranged in various ways. For a *bipolar bath* the limb is immersed in water in which are placed two electrodes, one at each end of the bath. The current has alternative pathways through the water and through the patient's tissues, so only a part of that applied passes through the tissues. Salt should not be added to the water, as it reduces its resistance and increases the proportion of the current that passes through it. Those muscles whose motor points are covered by the water are stimulated and the contractions obtained may be modified by altering the position of the electrodes. If, in a bipolar arm bath, the electrodes are placed opposite to the dorsal aspect of the limb, the extensor muscles contract rather than the flexors, while if they are opposite the ventral aspect the flexors contract most strongly.

In a *monopolar bath* one electrode is placed in the bath opposite to the distal part of the limb and the circuit completed either by a second monopolar bath or by a pad and electrode. In the bath some current passes through the water and some through the patient's tissues, but above the waterline all must pass through the tissues. There is stimulation of the muscles whose motor points are covered by the water and also possibly of other muscles in the pathway of the current. As with bipolar baths, it is possible to modify the effect by altering the position of the electrodes in the bath. The current that passes through the water enters the tissues at the waterline and its concentration in this area is liable to cause discomfort. This effect can be reduced by smearing an irregular line of petroleum jelly round the limb at the waterline, so increasing the length of the line along which current enters the tissues. Salt should not as a rule be added to the water as by reducing its resistance it increases the tendency for concentration of current at the waterline. Sometimes the resistance is too high for the output of the apparatus, and then a little salt may be used.

Although bath treatments are not commonly satisfactory when a localised effect is required, bipolar *faradic foot baths* are of value in the treatment of flat foot, and the application may be arranged in various ways. One method suitable for the stimulation of the muscles of the longitudinal arch is to place two electrodes transversely across the bottom of the bath, one under the heels and the other under the anterior part of the feet. The muscles of the anterior transverse arch may be stimulated by placing the electrodes one on each side of the feet, level with the metatarsal shafts, and with the ends of the electrodes just under the lateral borders of the feet. In both cases the water in the bath should just cover the toes. An alternative method of treatment is to place one electrode under the heels and to hold the other opposite to the motor points of the various muscles so that they are stimulated individually.

FARADISM OR SINUSOIDAL UNDER PRESSURE. This method is used to increase the venous and lymphatic drainage from an œdematous area. Contractions of many muscles are required, and may be obtained either by placing large pads so that they cover the motor points of the main muscle groups, or by the nerve conduction method. For the latter the main nerve trunks supplying the limb are stimulated above the œdematous area. The limb is supported in elevation, so that gravity assists the venous and lymphatic return, and is encased in an elastic bandage, which is most effective if applied over a thick layer of brown wool. The bandage increases the pressure on the vessels when the muscles contract, and its recoil on muscle relaxation exerts a further pumping action. The current is applied, and surged fairly slowly, in order to obtain a good pumping effect. Either the faradic or the sinusoidal current may be used, although the former is the more comfortable. The treatment lasts up to 20 minutes, but frequent rests should be given as it is somewhat fatiguing.

15

THE MODIFIED DIRECT CURRENT

Modifications of the Direct Current

INTERRUPTED DIRECT CURRENT. Interruption is
the most usual modification of the direct current, the flow of
current commencing and ceasing at regular intervals. The rise
and fall of intensity may be sudden, as in rectangular impulses
or gradual, as in trapezoidal, triangular and saw-tooth impulses (Fig. 92, page 124). The impulses in which the current
rises gradually are often termed selective, the reasons for this
being given below. The duration and frequency of the impulses
can be adjusted, a duration of 100 milliseconds sometimes being
used, although it is often an advantage to increase this to 300
or 600 milliseconds. When the duration of the impulses is
100 milliseconds the average frequency is 30 per minute, but if
the duration is increased the frequency must be reduced. In
some cases there is a reverse wave of current of low intensity
between the impulses, which are then said to be depolarised
(Fig. 92 (5)). This reduces the chemical actions at the electrodes. The resulting current is alternating, but the therapeutic
effects are the same as those of the interrupted direct current.

SURGED DIRECT CURRENT. The direct current is
occasionally surged, the intensity usually increasing gradually
and falling suddenly. If the surging is fairly rapid the resulting
current is similar to the saw-tooth impulses mentioned above.
Occasionally a slower rate of surging is used, each rise and
fall of current lasting for 1 second or more, and the current
may be reversed during alternate surges. Its graph is then
somewhat similar to that of the sinusoidal current although its
frequency is very much lower. A current of this type may be
referred to as "slow sinusoidal".

Physiological Effects

STIMULATION OF SENSORY NERVES. When the interrupted D.C. is applied to the body there is stimulation of the sensory nerves. The impulses are of fairly long duration, so the effect is rather marked, giving rise to a stabbing or burning sensation. There is reflex dilatation of the superficial blood vessels, and so erythema of the skin.

STIMULATION OF MOTOR NERVES. When a motor nerve is stimulated with the interrupted D.C., contraction of the muscles that it supplies is produced. The stimuli are infrequently repeated, so each one produces a brisk muscle twitch, followed by immediate relaxation. These isolated contractions have little beneficial effect on the muscles. When the current rises slowly a greater intensity is required to produce a muscle contraction than when it rises suddenly, because there is accommodation of the nerves (Chapter 13). A current that rises very slowly does not produce a muscle contraction.

STIMULATION OF DENERVATED MUSCLE. The interrupted direct current is capable of producing contractions of denervated muscle, provided that the intensity of current and duration of impulses are adequate. The contractions are sluggish in nature, the contraction and relaxation being slower than when the motor nerve is stimulated. As denervated muscle tissue has not the same property of accommodation as the motor nerves, a current that rises fairly slowly in intensity is as effective as one that rises suddenly. With the slowly rising current a contraction of denervated muscle can often be produced with an intensity of current that is insufficient to stimulate the motor nerves, and for this reason the impulses in which the current rises slowly are often termed selective. An impulse with a duration of 100 milliseconds is the shortest that is generally considered satisfactory for the treatment of denervated muscle, and it is often necessary to increase this in order to eliminate contractions of innervated muscles.

POLE USED FOR STIMULATING. The cathode is more effective than the anode for the stimulation of motor nerves, but when a muscle is denervated a better contraction is often produced with the anode than with the cathode. The reason for this is not known, and it does not always occur.

CHEMICAL EFFECTS. On the passage of a direct current through an electrolyte, chemical changes take place at the electrodes, so with the varied D.C. there is a danger of chemical burns, although this is less with a modified than with a constant D.C. When depolarised impulses are used, the reverse wave of current between the impulses reduces the chemical formation, and if the reverse wave is equal to the forward one any chemicals formed are neutralised and the danger of burns eliminated. In some cases the reverse wave is less than the forward one, and then there is some chemical formation, though less than with the direct current. This would occur with the current shown in Fig. 92 (5) on page 124. The reverse wave of current is of lower intensity than the forward wave and, as the durations of the two are the same, would not effect complete depolarisation. In practice the intervals are usually of longer duration than the impulses, so a reverse current of low intensity is adequate. Reduction of chemical formation has the additional advantage that it lessens the irritation of the skin.

Therapeutic Effects and Uses

The modified D.C. is not used in the treatment of normally innervated muscles, as the contractions produced by the surged faradic and sinusoidal currents are more like voluntary contractions, and so have greater beneficial effects than the isolated twitches produced by the modified D.C.

The main value of the modified D.C. lies in its property of producing contractions of denervated muscles. When a muscle is deprived of its nerve supply, changes in its structure and properties tend to occur. There is marked wasting of the muscle fibres and, if the denervation is longstanding, they tend to become fibrosed and to lose their properties of irritability, contractability, extensibility and elasticity. Electrical stimulation of the muscle fibres retards the development of these changes, although it is doubtful whether it is possible to restore the properties or muscle bulk by this means once they have been

lost. It is the only method by which contraction of the denervated fibres can be produced and it is probable that the contractions are of value in maintaining the vascularity of the
muscle and so retarding degeneration of the fibres. The stimulation must be strong enough to produce a muscle contraction,
and an adequate number of contractions must be produced.
Three hundred contractions of each muscle are desirable at each
treatment, although this is not always possible, either because
the muscle becomes fatigued or because, if many muscles are
affected, the duration of the treatment would be excessive.
Ninety is usually regarded as the minimum number of contractions to be effective, though if fatigue occurs before this number
is reached the treatment should be limited to a shorter duration.
Thus the modified D.C. is used in the treatment of lower motor
neurone lesions in which degeneration of the nerve fibres has
taken place. Its purpose is to maintain the muscle fibres in as
good a condition as possible until such time as re-innervation
of the muscle takes place. There is no object in using electrical
stimulation unless restoration of the nerve supply is anticipated,
or after a good active contraction has been re-established.

Choice of Current

TYPE OF IMPULSE. If a good muscle contraction is
obtained with a rectangular impulse, this may be used, but the
selective impulses often prove more satisfactory. The difference
between the various types of impulse lies in the time taken
for the intensity of current to rise to maximum. With the
rectangular impulses the rise is sudden, with the trapezoidal
it is fairly slow, with the triangular slower and with the saw-
tooth slower still, provided that the impulses are of the same
duration. The slow rise in the intensity of current has the
advantages that a contraction of denervated muscle is often
obtained with less sensory stimulation than when rectangular
impulses are used, and that denervated muscle often responds
to a lower intensity of current than that required to stimulate
motor nerves, so unwanted contractions of normally innervated
muscles in the region can be eliminated. In longstanding
denervation a muscle contraction may be obtained with a

current which rises slowly in intensity when there is no longer response to a rectangular impulse.

When various types of impulse are available it is advisable to attempt stimulation with each in order to ascertain which produces the most satisfactory contraction. It is often found that the more longstanding the denervation the slower the rise in intensity of current that is required.

DURATION OF IMPULSE. An impulse of at least 100 milliseconds is necessary in order to ensure that all the denervated muscle fibres are stimulated. If shorter impulses are used some of the muscle fibres may contract while others fail to do so. When attempting to eliminate contractions of normally innervated muscles, or to stimulate a muscle which has been denervated for some time, it is usually necessary to increase the duration of the impulses to 300 or 600 milliseconds.

SURGED D.C. A D.C. which is surged fairly quickly can be used instead of the selective impulses, though it usually proves less comfortable for the patient.

The slowly surged and reversed D.C. (slow sinusoidal) is rarely used. It has been claimed that it is capable of stimulating unstriped muscle tissue, but no proof of this is available. When considering this property the current must not be confused with the more rapidly varying sinusoidal current, the stimuli of which are much too brief to stimulate unstriped muscle tissue.

Methods of Application

When applying the modified D.C., the aim of treatment is direct stimulation of the muscle fibres. Therefore the treatment must be arranged so that the current passes through all the fibres of the muscle. There are various methods of achieving this.

One pad may be fixed over the origin of the muscle group, and each muscle stimulated in turn. The active electrode is a disc or small pad, which is either held over the lower end of the fleshy belly of the muscle to be stimulated, or stroked slowly down it. Moving the electrode over the muscle ensures that the current passes through a maximum number of fibres, also there is less irritation of the skin than when the active electrode is held in the same position throughout. These methods have the advantages that the current can be regulated to produce the optimum contraction of each muscle, and that each muscle is rested while other muscles of the group are being stimulated. It has the disadvantage that if there are many muscles to be stimulated it is not practicable to produce a large number of contractions of each.

Two disc electrodes may be used, one placed over each end of the muscle to be stimulated. This method is useful for the stimulation of deeply placed muscles, which are difficult to isolate, such as the extensor pollicis longus, but it is difficult to hold both electrodes and at the same time regulate the current intensity.

Two pads may be fixed, one over the origin and the other over the lower end of the muscle group to be stimulated. Provided that all the muscles contract equally, this method has the advantage that it permits a large number of contractions to be elicited. Great care must be taken that all the muscles contract satisfactorily. There may be a tendency for current to leak on to surrounding innervated muscles, but their contraction can usually be eliminated by the use of selective impulses of adequate duration.

It may be most convenient to apply an active pad which completely covers the muscle or group of muscles to be stimulated, the circuit being completed with a large directing or indifferent electrode. This method is satisfactory, for example, for the muscles of the shoulder girdle, when an indifferent electrode can be placed on the upper part of the anterior chest wall and a pad and plate electrode held over each of the muscles in turn.

The current could be applied in a bath, but this method is rarely satisfactory. The strongest muscles contract most easily, and it is usually impossible to produce adequate contractions of the weaker and more deeply placed muscles.

If no source of modified D.C. is available a constant current may be used, and the active electrode stroked rapidly over each muscle in turn. The muscle fibres are stimulated as the electrode passes over them. This method is liable to cause more discomfort and irritation of the skin than the preceding ones, and the stroking must be firm, rapid and rhythmical.

Technique

PREPARATION OF EQUIPMENT. The electronic apparatus is the most satisfactory, but if this is not available any source of constant D.C. can be used, and the current interrupted by moving the active electrode, as mentioned above. The apparatus is tested and other equipment prepared as for the treatmen s previously described. If a direct current is being used, without the reverse wave of current between the impulses, chemicals will be formed at the electrodes. In order to prevent these from reaching the skin, pads and coverings of disc electrodes must be of adequate thickness, at least eight layers of lint being advisable. No metal should be allowed to come in contact with the patient's tissues.

PREPARATION OF THE PATIENT. The skin is prepared by washing and protecting abrasions, as for other electrical treatments. It is often an advantage to soak the part in warm water before the treatment, to lower the resistance of the skin and to warm the muscles, although if there is extensive loss of sensation, care must be taken that the water is not too hot.

Contractions are obtained most easily if the part is supported so that the muscles to be stimulated are in a shortened position. Alternatively the current may be applied with the muscles in a partly lengthened position. This should only be done if the contractions produced are sufficiently strong to cause shortening of the muscle and so joint movement. If this is achieved the load opposing the muscle action should increase the beneficial effects. It is usually possible to produce movement only of the smaller joints, *e.g.* the wrist, although movement of the larger ones may be obtained if the limb is supported in slings.

APPLICATION OF CURRENT. Muscle contractions are often obtained most easily if the active electrode is connected to the anode, but this is not always the case. Each patient should be tested to determine whether the anode or the cathode produces the better response, and this pole used for the active electrode.

When the electrodes have been applied in one of the ways previously considered, the intensity of current is increased until a good muscle contraction is obtained. A large number of contractions is desirable, but any signs of fatigue, such as weakening of the contraction, are an indication for limiting the length of the treatment. The contractions are usually divided into groups, allowing rest periods between.

FREQUENCY OF TREATMENT. To be effective in retarding atrophy and maintaining the properties of the muscle tissue the current must be applied at frequent intervals and an adequate number of contractions elicited at each session. Daily treatment would be most satisfactory for the effects on the muscles, but the skin will rarely tolerate this. Usually treatment is given on 5 or 6 days a week. Great care must be taken to avoid the skin breaking down. It should be washed after treatment, and either powder or a soothing cream applied.

16

ELECTRICAL REACTIONS

Changes in Electrical Reactions

WHEN there is disease or injury of motor nerves or muscles, alterations are liable to occur in their response to electrical stimulation. The altered electrical reactions may be of considerable assistance in diagnosis of the type and extent of the lesion.

Reduction or loss of voluntary power of a muscle may be due to a lesion of the upper motor neurone, of the lower motor neurone, or of the muscle itself, the fault may be at the neuromuscular junction, or the disorder may be functional. The parts of the motor pathway which are normally accessible for electrical stimulation are the lower motor neurone below its exit from the vertebral canal, and the muscle itself, but not the anterior horn cell or the upper motor neurone.

UPPER MOTOR NEURONE LESIONS. When there is a lesion of the upper motor neurone, there are no changes in the lower motor neurone or muscle (*i.e.* in the accessible part of the motor pathway) which would lead to altered electrical reactions. Consequently a normal type of response is obtained, although sometimes the nerve and muscle are hyperexcitable and react to a lower intensity of current than that normally required.

LOWER MOTOR NEURONE LESIONS. Damage to a lower motor neurone may involve either the anterior horn cell or the fibres of the nerve roots or peripheral nerves. Lesions involving the nerve fibres can be divided into three groups:

(1) *Neurapraxia.* Bruising or pressure may render the nerve incapable of conducting impulses past the site of the lesion, and yet not be severe enough to cause degeneration of the fibres, the condition being known as neurapraxia. If the electrical

reactions are tested on the affected muscles a normal type of response is obtained, but there is loss of response to a stimulus applied to the nerve trunk above the lesion.

(2) *Axonotmesis* is liable to occur if the lesion is more severe. Degeneration of the axons takes place, the sheath of the nerve remaining intact, and this type of lesion may be observed in, for example, a radial nerve palsy associated with fractured shaft of the humerus. Once the nerve fibres have degenerated alterations in the electrical reactions occur.

(3) *Neurotmesis* is severing of the nerve sheath and fibres. The fibres degenerate below the site of the lesion, causing the same alterations in the electrical reactions as axonotmesis. The condition is, however, more serious, as suture of the nerve is necessary before satisfactory regeneration of the nerve can take place. A lesion of this type would be observed if, for example, the ulnar nerve were severed by a cut on the front of the wrist.

All these types of nerve lesion may be partial or complete, or there may be a mixture of two of them, *e.g.* neurapraxia and axonotmesis. If all the nerve fibres supplying a muscle degenerate, the reaction of complete denervation is observed, while if only some of the fibres degenerate the reaction is that of partial denervation.

The reactions observed in lesions of the *anterior horn cells* depend on the extent of the damage. If the severity of the lesion is such that there is degeneration of the nerve fibres, reaction of denervation is observed. If all the nerve cells supplying a muscle are affected, the reaction is that of complete denervation, while if only a proportion of the cells are involved, the reaction is that of partial denervation. In less severe lesions degeneration of the nerve fibres does not occur, and the reactions are normal.

NEUROMUSCULAR JUNCTION. Occasionally, as in the disease myasthenia gravis, reduction of voluntary power is due to faulty conduction at the neuromuscular junction. Methods other than electrical stimulation provide the most satisfactory aids to diagnosis of this condition.

MUSCLE LESIONS. If reduction of voluntary power is due to weakness or disease of the muscle, and there is no degeneration of the motor nerve, the electrical reactions are of normal type, but are reduced in strength. Should the lesion be so severe that there is complete loss of muscle tissue, there cannot be any response to electrical stimulation. This absence of response may occur in such conditions as ischaemic contracture or in the advanced stages of the myopathies, or may be due to fibrosis of muscles in longstanding denervation.

FUNCTIONAL DISORDERS. Loss of voluntary power may be due to hysterical paralysis, in which case there is no alteration in the electrical reactions.

DEVELOPMENT OF REACTION OF DENERVATION. When a nerve fibre is severed, Wallerian degeneration takes place below the site of the lesion, and above it as far as the first node of Ranvier. These changes may take up to fourteen days to become complete. If the nerve is stimulated below the site of the lesion, before degeneration has taken place, an impulse is initiated and a normal response of the muscle produced. Because of this, it may not be possible to make a full assessment of the lesion until three weeks after a suspected nerve injury, by which time any nerve fibres that have been severed will have degenerated. Tests carried out before this date can, however, provide useful information.

If a normal motor nerve trunk is stimulated with a current of adequate intensity, there is contraction of all the muscles it supplies beyond the point of stimulation. If, however, there is degeneration of the nerve fibres this response is reduced or lost, and the changes become evident three or four days after the injury. Changes in the reactions obtained on stimulation over the muscles may be observed before the end of one week, and indicate that the nerve is degenerating, although the ultimate extent of the degeneration cannot, at this stage, be assessed. Reaction of partial denervation would show that some of the nerve fibres had degenerated, but would not indicate how many more were still in the process of degeneration, or whether the denervation would ultimately become complete. If, however, the reaction of complete denervation were obtained, the severity of the lesion would immediately be apparent.

Strength-duration Curves

The plotting of strength-duration curves is the most satisfactory method at present available for the routine testing of electrical reactions in peripheral nerve lesions.

APPARATUS. The apparatus used for plotting strength-duration curves supplies rectangular impulses of different durations. Both the form and the durations of the impulses must be accurate, so it is necessary to use a stimulator specially designed for muscle testing. Impulses with durations of 0·01, 0·03, 0·1, 0·3, 1, 3, 10, 30 and 100 milliseconds are required, and the apparatus should be checked at regular intervals to ensure satisfactory working.

The stimulator may be of either the constant current or the constant voltage type. The differences between these two types of stimulator are beyond the scope of this book, but the former records the intensity of current used, the latter the voltage. Recent work indicates that the differences in the results obtained with the two types of stimulator have in the past been overestimated. The constant current stimulator was thought to produce the more accurate results, but the constant voltage stimulator is rather more comfortable for the patient.

METHOD. Before applying the current, the skin resistance is reduced by the methods used prior to other muscle stimulation, and the patient must be warm, fully supported and in a good light. An indifferent electrode may be applied to some convenient area, usually on the midline of the body or over the origin if the muscle group, and the active electrode over the fleshy part of the muscle, or two small electrodes may be used, one over each end of the muscle belly. In either case the active electrodes should be fairly small, in order that the muscles may be isolated from each other.

Current is applied, using the longest stimulus first, and increased until a minimal contraction is obtained. This may be assessed visually or by palpation of the tendon, depending on the muscle being tested. The intensity of the current (or voltage) is noted and the impulse shortened. This procedure is repeated with each stimulus in turn, the intensity of current

H

being increased as required. Utmost precision is essential if the results are to be accurate. A minimal contraction is used, as this makes it easy to detect any change in strength, and it is important that the active electrode is held on the same point over the muscle throughout the test.

The strength-duration curve is plotted from the results of the test, and although it will be further to the left with the constant

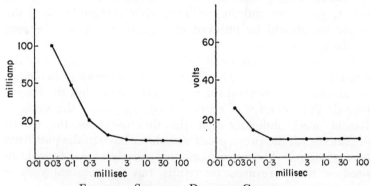

FIG. 122.—STRENGTH–DURATION CURVES OF
NORMALLY INNERVATED MUSCLE.

voltage than with the constant current stimulator, it is the shape of the curve that is the essential feature.

NORMAL INNERVATION. When all the nerve fibres supplying the muscle are intact, the strength-duration curve is that of normally innervated muscle (Fig. 122). The curve is of this typical shape because the impulses of longer durations all produce a response with the same strength of stimulus, irrespective of their duration, while those of shorter durations require an increase in the strength of the stimulus each time the duration is reduced. The reasons for this are given in Chapter 13. The point at which the curve begins to rise is variable, but is usually at a duration of impulse of 1 millisecond with the constant current and 0·1 millisecond with the constant voltage stimulator.

COMPLETE DENERVATION. When all the nerve fibres supplying a muscle have degenerated, the strength-duration curve is that of complete denervation (Fig. 123). When the duration of the impulse is 100 milliseconds or less, the strength of the stimulus must be increased each time the duration is reduced, and no response is obtained to the impulses of very

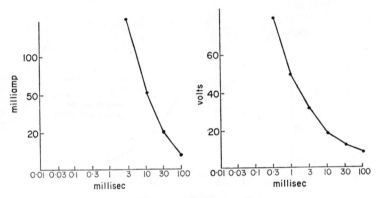

FIG. 123.—STRENGTH–DURATION CURVES OF
COMPLETELY DENERVATED MUSCLE.

short duration, so the curve rises steeply and is further to the right than that of normally innervated muscle.

PARTIAL DENERVATION. When some of the nerve fibres supplying a muscle have degenerated, while others are intact, the curve obtained is that of partial denervation (Fig. 124). The impulses of longer durations can stimulate both innervated and denervated muscle fibres, so a contraction is obtained with a stimulus of low intensity. As the impulses are shortened the denervated fibres respond less readily, a stronger stimulus is required to produce a perceptible contraction and the curve rises steeply like that of denervated muscle. With the impulses of shorter durations the innervated fibres respond to a weaker stimulus than that required for the denervated fibres, so contraction of the latter is not obtained and this part of the curve is similar to that of innervated muscle. Thus the right-hand part of the curve resembles that of denervated muscle, the left-hand part that of innervated muscle, and a kink is seen at the point where the two sections meet.

The shape of the curve indicates the proportion of denervation. If a large number of fibres are denervated the curve rises steeply and the greater part of it resembles that of denervation

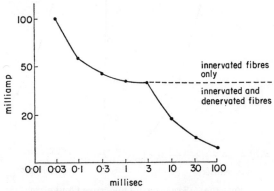

FIG. 124.—STRENGTH–DURATION CURVE OF
PARTIALLY DENERVATED MUSCLE.

(Fig. 125, a). If the majority of the fibres are innervated, the curve is lower and flatter and bears a closer resemblance to that of full innervation (Fig. 125, b).

An early sign of restoration of the nerve supply to a muscle may be changes in the shape of the strength-duration curve. A kink appears in the curve and, as re-innervation progresses, the curve moves down and to the left. Progressive denervation is indicated by the appearance of a kink, increase in the slope and shift of the curve to the right.

The advantages of this method of testing electrical reactions are that it is simple and reliable and indicates the proportion of denervation, while a series of tests shows changes in the condition. Its disadvantages are that in large muscles only a proportion of the fibres may respond, so that the full picture is not clearly shown, and that it does not indicate the site of the nerve lesion. The latter may be remedied by testing nerve conduction.

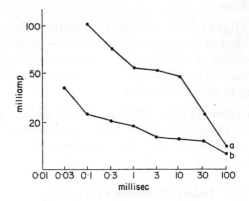

FIG. 125.—STRENGTH–DURATION CURVES OF PARTIALLY DENERVATED MUSCLE, SHOWING DIFFERENT DEGREES OF DENERVATION.

Nerve Conduction Tests

NERVE CONDUCTIVITY. Stimulation of a nerve trunk causes contraction of the muscles supplied by that nerve distal to the point of stimulation, and testing of nerve conduction is commonly used in conjunction with the plotting of strength-duration curves. An impulse with a duration of 0·1 or 0·3 millisecond is applied at a point where the nerve trunk is superficial, and any contraction of the muscles supplied below this point indicates that at least some of the nerve fibres are intact. Comparison with the strength of the stimulus required to produce a similar reaction on the unaffected side of the body gives some indication of the severity of the lesion, although it does not show whether the fault lies in the nerve or in the muscle itself.

When a nerve fibre is degenerating, conductivity is lost distal to the lesion within a few days, and this can give some indication of the state of the lesion and possible prognosis at a date earlier than that at which the full test can accurately be performed.

In lesions in which degeneration does not occur, it may be

possible to determine the level at which the impulses are blocked by testing at different points on the nerve trunk. Stimulation below, but not above the site of the lesion, should elicit a response.

NERVE DISTRIBUTION. The distribution of the different nerves is subject to some variation, which may prove misleading in the assessment of nerve lesions. The distribution of a nerve can be determined by stimulating the nerve trunk and observing the resulting muscle contractions.

CONDUCTION SPEED. The speed with which an impulse is transmitted along a nerve fibre can be measured with suitable equipment, and this is considered in the section on electromyography (below).

Other Methods of Testing

Various other methods of testing electrical reactions have been used. The principles of some of these are given below, and the reasons that their results are not satisfactory.

RHEOBASE. This is the smallest intensity of current that will produce a muscle contraction if the stimulus is of infinite duration, an impulse of 100 milliseconds being used in practice. In denervation the rheobase may be less than that of innervated muscle, and often rises as re-innervation commences. These factors are not, however, sufficiently constant to be reliable guides. The rheobase varies considerably in different muscles and according to the skin resistance and temperature of the part, while a rise may be due to fibrosis of the muscle.

CHRONAXIE. This is the duration of the shortest impulse that will produce a response with a current of double the rheobase. The chronaxie of innervated muscle is appreciably less than that of denervated muscle, the former being less and the latter more than 1 millisecond if the constant voltage stimulator is used. With the constant current stimulator the values are higher, but bear a similar relationship to each other. Chronaxie is not a satisfactory method of testing electrical reactions, as partial denervation is not clearly shown, the chronaxie being that of the predominant fibres, *e.g.* the

chronaxie of a muscle with 25 per cent of its fibres innervated would be the same as that of a completely denervated
muscle.

PULSE RATIO. This is the ratio of the current needed to
produce a muscle contraction with an impulse of 1 millisecond
to that required if the duration of the impulse is 100 milliseconds. With innervated muscle little or no increase in the
intensity of current is necessary when the impulse is shortened
from 100 to 1 millisecond, so the pulse ratio is low, less than
2·2. Denervated muscle requires a greater increase in the
intensity of current, so the pulse ratio is higher, usually more
than 2·5. The disadvantages of this method are the same as
those of chronaxie, in that partial denervation is not clearly
shown.

FARADIC–I.D.C. TEST. The method of testing with the
faradic and interrupted direct currents was widely used in the
past, but it is very inaccurate.

The faradic current provides impulses with a duration of
0·1 to 1 millisecond and a frequency of 50–100 per second.
These cause a tetanic contraction of innervated muscle, but
with a faradic coil it is difficult or impossible to elicit a response
from denervated muscle, owing to the short duration of the
stimuli. With modern stimulators, however, a response of
denervated muscle can usually be obtained with impulses of
this duration, owing to the greater output and more comfortable
current than that provided by the older equipment. Further
inaccuracies arose with the latter because the form and duration
of the impulses varied with currents from different sources.

The interrupted direct current provides impulses with a
duration of approximately 100 milliseconds, repeated 30 times
per minute. These usually produce a brisk contraction of
innervated muscle fibres, but a sluggish contraction of denervated fibres. Innervated muscles may, however, respond
sluggishly if their temperature is below normal, and in certain
other conditions, such as myxoedema, while the contraction
of denervated muscle becomes brisker as its temperature
rises.

Electromyography

Electromyography is the study of the electrical activity in muscle tissue, some examples of which are given below.

METHOD. The usual method is to use a needle electrode inserted into the muscle. This may be bipolar, consisting of two electrodes, one lying within but insulated from the other, or monopolar, with a second electrode on the surface of the body. Sometimes two small electrodes are placed on the skin over the muscle, but this method is less accurate. A circuit is completed between the two electrodes and any current flowing

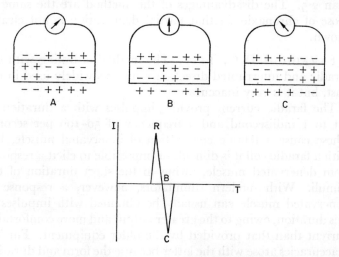

FIG. 126.—PRODUCTION OF AN ACTION POTENTIAL.

in the circuit is amplified, led to a loud speaker and cathode ray tube, where the graph of the current is seen on the screen.

ACTION POTENTIALS. When a muscle fibre is inactive a potential difference exists across its plasma membrane, the outer surface bearing a positive and the inner surface a negative charge. As the fibre contracts a wave of reversal of polarity passes along it, and if a circuit is completed between its ends current flows first in one direction then in the other, giving a diphasic action potential (Fig. 126).

INTERFERENCE PATTERNS. Normal muscle at rest shows no electrical activity, but action potentials are produced on contraction. Each motor unit sets up its own action potentials, but those from the different motor units are not synchronous and appear one after the other in an irregular manner. This produces an interference pattern on the screen and a low rumble, or, with greater activity, a loud roar on the loud speaker.

FIBRILLATION POTENTIALS. When a muscle is deprived of its nerve supply spontaneous contraction of individual muscle fibres is liable to occur. This is termed fibrillation and produces potentials of shorter duration and lower amplitude than normal action potentials. These appear as diphasic spikes on the screen and produce sharp clicks on the loud speaker.

POLYPHASIC UNITS. When motor units are incompletely innervated, polyphasic potentials are produced on attempted muscle contraction. These are observed in the early stages of re-innervation of a muscle, but may also occur when the nerve is degenerating in a neuropathy.

VALUE OF ELECTROMYOGRAPHY. Evidence provided by electromyography is of assistance in differentiating between lesions of the anterior horn cells, the nerve fibres and the muscles, and typical electrical activity observed in conditions such as the myopathies and myasthenia gravis may prove an aid to diagnosis. Interpretation of the findings of electromyography does, however, require considerable knowledge and experience, and is the field of the physician, not that of the physiotherapist.

In peripheral nerve lesions electromyography used in conjunction with the plotting of strength-duration curves may be of assistance in assessing the lesion. Minimal innervation may be detected by the appearance of normal action potentials at a stage when no other signs of innervation are present, while fibrillation potentials are a definite sign of denervation.

Electromyography is also used in the measurement of nerve conduction velocities, considered below.

In addition to its use as a diagnostic agent, electromyography is of assistance in determining the actions of normal muscles and in analysing the muscle work involved in performing complex movements.

NERVE CONDUCTION VELOCITY. Stimulation of a motor nerve trunk elicits a contraction of the muscles which it supplies, and the speed with which the nerve impulse travels can be assessed by measuring the interval that elapses between the application of the stimulus and the resulting action potential in a muscle. This, considered relative to the distance from the point of stimulation to the muscle, gives the velocity of the nerve impulse.

Reduced rate of conduction occurs if there is reduction in the calibre of the nerve fibres, as may be caused by pressure, and so indicates the nature and severity of the lesion. In median carpal tunnel syndrome, reduction in the rate of conduction of the median nerve is apparent if the nerve is stimulated at the front of the wrist and the time required for an impulse to reach the abductor pollicis brevis muscle measured. The site of a nerve lesion may be determined by measuring the conduction velocity over different stretches of a nerve. Reduced rate of transmission in one section indicates that this is the area in which the fault lies.

The conduction velocity of sensory nerves can also be measured. When the nerve is stimulated distally, the potentials produced by the nerve impulses can be detected at more proximal points where the nerve trunk is superficial. This may be of assistance in assessing a lesion in which sensory fibres are involved, such as an ulnar neuritis.

PART II

ELECTROTHERAPY—HIGH-FREQUENCY CURRENTS

17

PHYSICS OF
HIGH-FREQUENCY CURRENTS

A HIGH-FREQUENCY current is a current which
alternates so rapidly that it does not stimulate motor or
sensory nerves. To achieve this it must have a frequency of
more than approximately 500,000 cycles per second, and it is
often termed an oscillating current.

Oscillations

Oscillation may be defined as a "swinging to and fro," and
oscillation of many different objects can be observed during
everyday activities, *e.g.* a swinging pendulum, a vibrating
piano string. A high-frequency alternating current is described
as an oscillating current, because the electrons swing to and fro
n the circuit, and the behaviour of an oscillating current
in many ways resembles that of other oscillating systems.

THE OSCILLATING SYSTEM. During any series of oscillations a certain sequence of events occurs, and a weight swinging
on the end of a string provides a simple example of these.
Before the oscillations can commence the weight must be
drawn to one side (Fig. 127A$_1$), that is, energy is supplied to
the system. When the weight has been drawn to one side,
but before it is released, the energy is in the form of potential
energy. When the weight is released, it swings down to the
vertical position, but the momentum it develops carries it
beyond the vertical (Fig. 127B$_1$). Throughout the movement
it has kinetic energy. When it reaches the limit of its swing it
pauses for an instant (Fig. 127C$_1$), and the energy is once again

potential. Then the weight swings in the reverse direction (Fig. 127D$_1$), and the sequence of events is repeated.

An oscillating current is produced by discharging a condenser through an inductance of low ohmic resistance (Chapter 6). The condenser must first be charged (Fig. 127A$_2$), *i.e.* energy is supplied to the circuit, the static charge on the condenser representing potential energy. The condenser then discharges through the circuit and as it does so the current sets up a self-induced EMF in the inductance. This EMF retards the rise of current and prolongs its flow when it is tending to fall

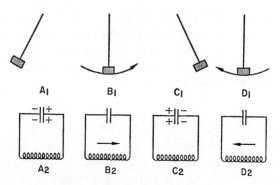

FIG. 127.—OSCILLATING SYSTEMS.

(Fig. 127B$_2$), the latter effect corresponding to the momentum of the weight in that it continues the movement after the neutral position has been reached. The current represents kinetic energy. The self-induced EMF which prolongs the flow of current recharges the condenser with the reverse polarity to its original charge (Fig. 127C$_2$) and the energy is once more potential. The condenser then discharges again, giving a flow of current in the reverse direction to the previous one (Fig. 127D$_2$), and the series of events is repeated.

FREQUENCY OF OSCILLATIONS. Each complete swing, *i.e.* from the starting point back to the same point, is one cycle of oscillation, and the frequency of the oscillations is the number of cycles in unit time.

When a weight is swinging on a string it oscillates at a

definite frequency, which depends on the length of the string. If the string is short the frequency is high, but as it is lengthened the frequency decreases, and in each case the weight will oscillate at a particular frequency, but at no other. Thus the frequency of the oscillations depends on the physical properties of the system and is a constant factor for any particular system. Similarly the frequency of an oscillating current depends on the properties of the circuit in which it is produced, being determined by the capacity of the condenser and the inductance of the coil. If the condenser has a small capacity it holds only a small quantity of electricity when charged to a given voltage. When it discharges this electricity soon passes round the circuit and the flow of current is of short duration. As each current flow lasts only for a short time, many occur in a given period and the frequency of the oscillations is high. If the inductance of the circuit is small, only a small self-induced EMF is set up; this does not retard the rise of current and prolong its flow to any great extent, so again each flow of current is of short duration and the frequency is high. The frequency can be calculated by the formula:

$$f = \frac{1}{2\pi \sqrt{LC}}$$

where f = number of cycles per second.
C = capacity of condenser, measured in farads.
L = inductance of circuit, measured in henries.

Thus the frequency of the oscillating current is inversely proportional to the product of the capacity of the condenser and the inductance of the circuit. Capacity and inductance are constant factors for any particular circuit, and so there is a particular frequency at which the current tends to oscillate in any circuit. This may be described as the natural frequency of the circuit.

DAMPING OF OSCILLATIONS. As the system oscillates energy is lost to the surrounding medium, and each excursion is less than the preceding one. This is known as damping of the oscillations. The rate at which the energy is lost depends on the amount of resistance that is offered to the movement.

If the weight is swinging in air, the air offers some resistance to the movement, and each swing is rather less than the preceding one. If it were swinging in some medium which offered more resistance, more energy would be lost and the damping would occur more rapidly.

When the condenser is discharging, the ohmic resistance of the circuit impedes the flow of current. If the ohmic resistance is low, little energy is lost during each flow of current and each oscillation is only a little less than the preceding one (Fig. 128A). If the ohmic resistance is high more energy is lost, the damping occurs more quickly (Fig. 128B) and the oscillations are said to be strongly damped.

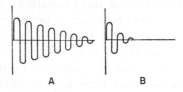

A   B

FIG. 128.—DAMPED OSCILLATIONS.

TRANSFER OF ENERGY BETWEEN OSCILLATING SYSTEMS. During the oscillation energy is lost to the surrounding medium, and causes a disturbance of this medium which is capable of influencing a second system situated in the region of the first. The swinging weight disturbs the air around it, and when the movement of the air set up by the first swing of the weight strikes the second system it causes the weight to swing to one side (Fig. 129). Energy has been supplied to the second system, which then tends to oscillate at a frequency determined by the length of its string. The first system, however, continues to oscillate at a frequency determined by the length of its string, and sets up in the air disturbances of the same frequency as the oscillations. Thus it continues to influence the second system. If the two tend to oscillate at the same frequency, the disturbances set up by one augment the oscillations of the other, and both continue to oscillate until all the energy has been lost to the surrounding medium. For this to occur the natural frequency must be the same for both and they are then said to be in tune, or in resonance, with each other. If the natural frequencies of the two systems are not the same, the disturbances set up by one tend to oppose the oscillation of the other and stop the movement.

This may be compared with a child swinging another child in a swing. The push forwards is given just as the swing commences its forward movement, and one push is applied for each complete forward and backward movement of the swing. This corresponds to systems in resonance, when the disturbance set up by one system has the same frequency as, and therefore augments, the movement of the other. If, on the other hand, three forward pushes are given at equal intervals during one

FIG. 129.—TRANSFER OF ENERGY BETWEEN OSCILLATING SYSTEMS.

complete forward and backward movement of the swing, the frequency of the pushes is not the same as that of the swing. The third forward push is applied as the swing is coming back, and so stops the movement. Similarly, if the disturbance set up by one system has not the same frequency as the movement of the other, it opposes the motions and stops the oscillation.

If a piano string and a violin string are tuned to the same pitch, striking the note on the piano causes the violin string to sound. The strings tend to vibrate at the same frequency, and the sound waves set up in the air by the piano string also have this frequency. When these strike the violin string they cause it to vibrate, as the strings are in resonance.

In a similar manner a current oscillating in one circuit can produce an oscillating current in a second circuit, provided that the second circuit is in tune, or in resonance, with the first. When an electric current oscillates it disturbs the ether and sets up wireless waves, which are one type of electromagnetic waves (Chapter 21). The wireless waves have the same frequency as the current which produces them, and when they strike a second circuit they tend to produce current in this circuit. This can be illustrated by considering the circuits shown in Fig. 130.

Current is oscillating in the transmitting circuit T at a frequency dependent upon the product of the capacity and the inductance of this circuit (C_1L_1). The current sets up wireless waves of the same frequency, which travel through the ether and strike the receiving circuit R. The first wireless wave to strike this circuit produces a current which charges the condenser. The condenser then discharges, setting up an oscillating current, the frequency of which depends on the product of the capacity and the inductance of the receiving circuit (C_2L_2). Wireless waves set up by the current in the transmitting circuit

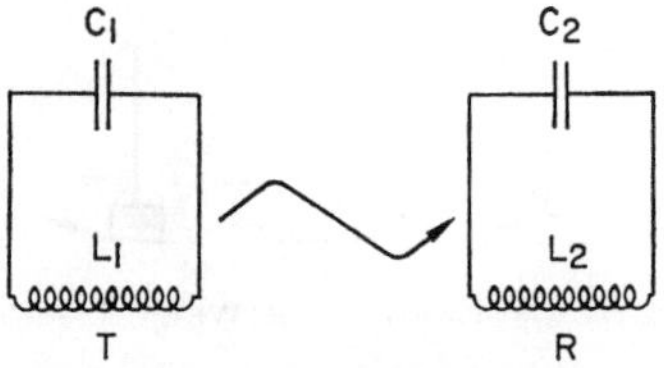

Fig. 130.—Transfer of Energy between Circuits.

continue to arrive and influence the receiving circuit. If the natural frequencies of the two circuits are the same, these wireless waves arrive at the right moment to augment the oscillations, but if the natural frequencies are different, they oppose and stop the oscillations. Thus, for current to be produced in the receiving circuit, the natural frequencies of this and the transmitting circuit must be the same, i.e. the product of capacity and inductance must be the same for both circuits $(C_1L_1 = C_2L_2)$. The circuits are then said to be in resonance.

A second circuit can be tuned to a transmitting circuit by altering either the capacity of a condenser or the length of a coil of wire in the circuit. When the product of the units of inductance of the coil and capacity of the condenser is the same for both circuits, then current oscillates at the same frequency in both. For instance, if one circuit has 3 units of capacity and 4 units of inductance, the product is 12 units. If another circuit has 2 units of capacity and 6 units of inductance, the product is again 12 units and the second circuit is in resonance with the first. With the short-wave diathermic machine a variable condenser is placed in the resonator circuit and this circuit is tuned to the oscillator circuit by altering the capacity of the condenser.

Properties of High-Frequency Currents

A high-frequency current has a frequency of more than approximately 500,000 cycles per second and does not stimulate motor or sensory nerves. The oscillations may be sustained or unsustained, damped or undamped.

SUSTAINED AND UNSUSTAINED OSCILLATIONS. When the oscillations of a high-frequency current follow each other

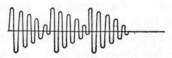

FIG. 131.—SUSTAINED OSCILLATIONS.

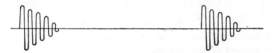

FIG. 132.—UNSUSTAINED OSCILLATIONS.

closely they are said to be sustained (Fig. 131), but when there is a pause between each group of oscillations they are described as unsustained (Fig. 132).

DAMPED AND UNDAMPED OSCILLATIONS. When the amplitude of each oscillation of the current is less than its

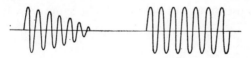

FIG. 133.—(A) DAMPED, (B) UNDAMPED OSCILLATIONS.

predecessor, the oscillations are said to be damped (Fig. 133(A)), but when the amplitude of all the oscillations is the same they are described as being undamped (Fig. 133(B)).

HEAT PRODUCTION. Heat is produced by a high-frequency current, as by other currents, in accordance with Joule's law.

IMPEDANCE. When the frequency of a current is high inductive reactance is considerable, and increases as the frequency increases (Chapter 5). Capacitive reactance, however, is not very great, and decreases as the frequency increases (Chapter 6). Thus the impedance offered to a high frequency current by an inductance in the circuit may be considerable, but that due to the presence of a condenser may be small, both effects being more apparent if the frequency is very high. Because of these properties a high frequency current behaves in a rather different manner from one of a lower frequency. The ohmic resistance of a circuit may appear to be less than that encountered by a low frequency current, as a thin layer of material of high resistance acts as the dielectric of a condenser, so offering much less impedance to the passage of a high than of a low frequency current.

ELECTROMAGNETIC WAVES. As the high-frequency current oscillates, electromagnetic waves are set up. These have the same frequency as the current, and are wireless, or Hertzian waves (Chapter 21).

MAGNETIC AND ELECTROSTATIC DISTURBANCES. When a high-frequency current flows in a circuit, it is found that at certain points (the antinodes of potential) an electrostatic field is set up, while at other points (the nodes of potential) a magnetic field is set up. This can be illustrated by comparison with water.

If the hand is moved to and fro in a bath of water, the water is made to oscillate, and behaves in the same way as any other

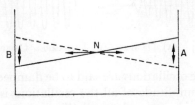

FIG. 134.—OSCILLATION OF WATER.

oscillating system. At one moment the level of the water is high at one end of the bath (Fig. 134, A), low at the other (Fig. 134, B), as shown by the continuous line in Fig. 134. The water then swings through N, the movement is prolonged by its momentum, and the level rises at B, falls at A, as shown by the dotted line in Fig. 134. The water pauses for an instant, then swings back again, and the oscillations continue. At A and B, which lie at the limits of the system, the level of the water changes and the energy is potential. These points are termed the antinodes. At N, which is in the centre of the system, the level does not change but the water moves to and fro and the energy is kinetic. This point is termed the node. It is found that in order to make the water oscillate the hand must be moved to and fro with a definite frequency, and that this frequency is dependent upon the size of the bath. Thus the system has a natural frequency at which the water tends to oscillate, and there is a relationship between this frequency and the size of the system.

If the hand is moved to and fro in a much larger expanse of water, $e.g.$ a pond, a similar to and fro movement of the water is produced, but spreads outwards as a series of waves. On observing the waves it is seen that although the waves appear to travel over the surface of the water, the water itself swings to and fro in a limited area, and does not travel from one place to another. An object floating on the surface of the water moves up and down, and to and fro within a limited area, but not from one part of the pond to another. As the hand is moved forward, the water is thrust in one direction, as it is moved back, the water is drawn back again, $i.e.$ the water in this area is made to oscillate. The force of the movement sets up a similar oscillation in the adjacent area, and so on in the next area, giving the appearance of a wave travelling over the surface as the water oscillates in one section after another. Thus the wave really consists of a series of oscillating systems lying end to end. In Fig. 135 the continuous line represents the surface of the water at one instant, the dotted line a moment later. The water swings to and fro in the sections A_1A_2, A_2A_3, etc., each of which represents a separate oscillating system. The points A_1, A_2, A_3 are the antinodes and are situated at the limits of the systems, where the level of the water changes and the energy is potential. The points N_1, N_2, etc., are the nodes, which lie in the centre of the systems where the water swings to and fro and the energy is kinetic. It can be seen from Fig. 135 that the distance between any two adjacent antinodes or nodes is equal to half the wave-length (wave-length is the distance from any point on one wave to the same point on the next wave), and that each oscillating system is equal in length to half the wave-length.

An oscillating current behaves in the same way as the water. In a simple system consisting of a condenser and a coil the

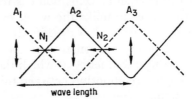

FIG. 135.—WAVES ON THE SURFACE OF WATER.

static charge on the condenser, which is potential energy, is produced at the limits of the pathway through which the electrons swing, and these points are the antinodes of potential. The current in the coil, which represents kinetic energy, flows through the centre of the system, and this point is the node of potential. The static charge at the antinodes of potential sets up an electrostatic field and the current at the node of potential sets up a magnetic field. Like the water, the circuit has a natural frequency at which the current tends to oscillate, and there is a definite relationship between the frequency and the length of the system. The distance between two adjacent antinodes is half the wave-length of the wireless waves which are set up by the current, and the system must be of this length for the current to oscillate in it.

If a longer circuit is considered it is found to consist of a series of such systems. When a rapidly varying EMF is applied, the electrons move first in one direction, pause for an instant as the EMF reverses, and then swing back again. So each group of electrons swings to and fro in a limited section of the wire. At the limits of each system the electrons pause for an instant before moving in the reverse direction, the energy is potential and an electrostatic field is set up. The electrons move through the centre of each section, the energy is kinetic and the current sets up a magnetic field. The points at which there is maximum potential energy are the antinodes of potential, those at which there is maximum current are the nodes of potential. As with the water, the distance between any two adjacent nodes or antinodes is equal to half the wave-length

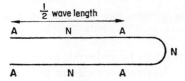

FIG. 136.—NODES AND ANTINODES OF A CIRCUIT.

of the wireless waves set up by the current (Fig. 136). Thus as the current flows a series of separate oscillating systems is set up, each of which is equal in length to half the wave-length of the wireless waves. The wave-length varies inversely with the frequency of the current, and so the higher the frequency the smaller is each of these systems and the nearer together are the nodes and antinodes. For current to flow in such a circuit, it must form a series of complete oscillating systems. The length of each system is half the wave-length of the wireless waves set up by the current, so the length of the circuit must be a multiple of this distance.

It has been seen that the current in any circuit tends to oscillate at a definite frequency, and that the circuit must be of a suitable length for the current to oscillate in it. When dealing with high-frequency generators, such as the short-wave diathermic machine, a current of a certain frequency is produced. In order that this current may flow in an external circuit connected to the machine, the circuit must be arranged in such a way that currents of this particular frequency can oscillate in it. The length of the cable electrode is usually equal to half the wave-length of the wireless waves set up by the current, so that it forms one complete oscillating system. When the cable is used the circuit is arranged so that the antinodes of potential lie at the ends of the cable, the node at the centre (Fig. 137). Thus an electrostatic field is set up between the ends of the cable, a magnetic field at its centre.

When the condenser electrodes are used the situation is different. Inclusion of a condenser in the circuit enables the

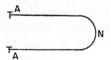

FIG. 137.—NODES AND ANTINODES OF THE CABLE
ELECTRODE.

length of the circuit to be reduced, as the condenser acts as a reservoir for the electrons, which are able to swing to and fro in a shorter circuit than would otherwise be required. The larger the condenser, the more can the circuit be shortened, but it must still be of a definite length, determined by the frequency of the current and the capacity of the condenser.

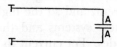

FIG. 138.—ANTINODES WITH THE CONDENSER ELECTRODES.

The length of the leads for the condenser electrodes varies for different machines, and for electrodes of different sizes, but unless the leads are of the correct length a satisfactory output is not obtained. When the condenser electrodes are used the arrangement of the circuit is such that the electrodes lie at the antinodes and an electrostatic field is set up between them (Fig. 138).

18

PRODUCTION OF
HIGH-FREQUENCY CURRENTS

Types of High Frequency Current

A SHORT-WAVE diathermic current has a frequency of between 10,000,000 and 100,000,000 cycles per second and sets up wireless waves with a wave-length of between 30 and 3 metres. Any current within this range is classed as short-wave diathermy, but that commonly used for medical work has a frequency of 27,120,000 cycles per second and sets up wireless waves with a wave-length of 11 metres. The long-wave diathermic current, which was used extensively in the past but has now largely been replaced by short-wave diathermy, has a frequency of approximately 1,000,000 cycles per second and sets up wireless waves with a wave-length of 300 metres. The currents are termed long- and short-wave diathermy on account of the relative wave-lengths of the wireless waves that they set up.

Principles of Production

It is not possible to construct any mechanical device which causes sufficiently rapid movement to produce a high-frequency current, so this type of current is obtained by discharging a condenser through an inductance of low ohmic resistance. The basic oscillator circuit consists of a condenser and an inductance, and currents of different frequencies are obtained by selecting suitable condensers and inductances. If a current of very high frequency is required, the capacity and inductance are small, while to produce a current of lower frequency a larger condenser and/or inductance are used.

In order to produce the high-frequency current the condenser must be made to charge and discharge repeatedly, and to achieve this the basic oscillator circuit is incorporated in either a spark-gap or a valve circuit, the latter being commonly used in apparatus encountered in the physiotherapy department.

The Valve Short-Wave Diathermic Machine

There are various circuits which may be used in valve diathermic machines. The example given below serves to illustrate the principles of working but it is considerably simpler than any which is actually employed.

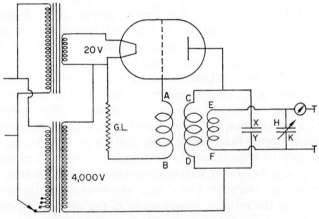

FIG. 139.—VALVE DIATHERMIC MACHINE.

CONSTRUCTION. (Fig. 139). The primary coils of two transformers are connected to a source of A.C. One is a step-down transformer, and its secondary coil supplies current to the filament heating circuit of a triode valve. The other is a step-up transformer and is connected to the anode circuit, which consists of the triode valve and the oscillator circuit, the latter comprising a condenser (XY) and the oscillator coil (CD). Another coil (AB) lies close to the oscillator coil and has one end connected to the grid of the triode valve, the other through the grid leak resistance (GL) to the filament of the valve. The patient's, or resonator, circuit consists of a coil (EF) lying close to the oscillator coil, and a variable condenser (HK), which is usually in parallel to the patient's terminals.

PRODUCTION OF THE OSCILLATING CURRENT. The A.C. from the source of supply passes through the primary coils of the transformers and EMFs are induced in the secondary coils. An EMF of 20 to 25 volts is set up in the secondary coil of the step-down transformer and produces current through the filament of the valve. The filament is heated, thermionic emission takes place and the valve becomes capable of conducting current. An EMF of about 4,000 volts is induced in

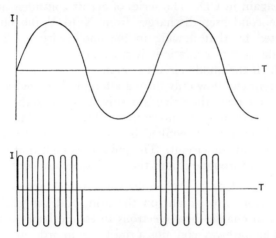

FIG. 140.—CURRENT IN SHORT-WAVE DIATHERMY MACHINE—
A.C. SUPPLY AND OSCILLATIONS PRODUCED.

the secondary coil of the step-up transformer and, provided that the polarity is such that the anode of the valve is positive relative to the filament, current flows in the anode circuit. The current passes from the transformer, across the valve, through the oscillator coil in the direction C to D, and back to the transformer. As the current in the oscillator coil rises in intensity, an EMF is induced in the coil AB, electrons moving from B to A. These electrons move on to the grid of the valve, giving it a negative charge which stops the flow of current in the anode circuit. As the intensity of the current in CD falls, self-induced EMF prolongs the current flow and charges the condenser XY with Y negative and X positive. When the self-induced EMF dies away the condenser discharges back through the oscillator coil, current flowing from D to C. As CD is an inductance, this is the first wave of an oscillating discharge and self-induced EMF recharges the condenser with X negative and Y positive. The flow of current from D to C induces an EMF in AB, electrons moving from A to B, so that the grid loses its negative charge and the anode current flows again. The next wave of the condenser discharge is now commencing, current flowing from X to Y, and this is augmented by the anode current flowing again in CD. The series of events continues and each time the condenser discharges from X to Y the current is augmented by that flowing in the anode circuit. Thus the amplitude of the oscillations is maintained and they are un-damped. If the anode circuit is supplied with A.C., as in Fig. 139, current can flow only during alternate half-cycles of A.C., when the anode of the valve is positive relative to the filament, and the oscillations are intermittent (Fig. 140). More usually the supply current is rectified by means of valves before it is taken to the anode circuit. The polarity is such that the valve can conduct throughout and the oscillations are continuous.

THE GRID LEAK. When the current flows across the valve some electrons are caught on the grid, and the grid leak is provided to enable these electrons to escape back to the fila-ment. The pathway contains a resistance in order to maintain a P.D. between the filament and the grid.

CURRENT SUPPLIED TO THE PATIENT. The resonator coil (EF) lies within the varying magnetic field set up around the oscillator coil, so, provided that the two circuits are in resonance, a high-frequency current is induced in it. This current is similar to that in the oscillator circuit and is supplied to the patient, the circuit being tuned by the variable condenser (HK).

THE VARIABLE CONDENSER. In order that current flowing in the oscillator circuit may produce a similar high-frequency current in the resonator circuit, the two circuits must be in resonance. That is, their natural frequencies must be the same, and to achieve this the product of inductance and capacity must be the same for both circuits. When short-wave diathermy is applied by the condenser field method, the electrodes and patient's tissues form a condenser, the capacity of which depends on the size of the electrodes and on the distance and material between them, and so is different for each application. When the cable electrode is used it forms an inductance, the value of which varies according to its arrangement. Consequently either the capacity or the inductance of the patient's circuit is varied at each treatment, and the variable condenser is essential to compensate for this. When the electrodes have been arranged in position, the capacity of the variable condenser is adjusted until the product of the inductance and capacity of the resonator circuit is equal to that in the oscillator circuit.

DETECTION OF TUNING. When the oscillator and resonator circuits are in tune with each other, the ammeter shows a maximum reading, the needle swinging back whichever way the knob controlling the variable condenser is turned. Tuning may also be detected by placing a tube containing a small amount of neon gas within the electric field between the electrodes or ends of the cable (see page 297). The gas within the tube glows at maximum intensity when the circuits are in resonance.

THE AMMETER. In Fig. 139 the meter is shown in the patient's circuit, but it may be situated in some other part of the machine. A meter in the patient's circuit does not register the current that the patient is receiving, only that which is charging the condenser of which the patient forms a part, or that which is flowing through the cable which is coiled in relationship to the patient's tissues. It is therefore impossible to calculate the intensity of current that should be applied for any particular treatment, although a record of the meter reading may be of value at subsequent treatments in indicating the current used previously. The main purpose of the meter is to show when the oscillator and resonator circuits are in tune with each other. When this is so maximum output is obtained from the machine, and this can be indicated by a meter placed in some other part of the circuit.

REGULATION OF CURRENT. When the machine is

switched on there may be slight delay before current flows in the anode circuit, as some machines incorporate a thermal delay switch which prevents the passage of current through this circuit until the filament of the valve reaches an adequate temperature. When current flows in the anode circuit, the resonator circuit is tuned in order that current may be obtained in it. The current is then increased to the required intensity by shortening the primary coil of the step-up transformer which supplies the anode circuit. This is done by moving a selector switch over studs, and each time the primary coil is shortened the difference in length between it and the secondary coil is increased. This increases the extent to which the voltage is stepped up, and as a greater voltage is applied to the anode circuit the intensity of the current is increased.

Methods of Current Regulation

There are various ways of regulating the intensity of current supplied to the patient from a short-wave diathermic machine, different methods being used in different models.

THE ANODE VOLTAGE. The current can be controlled by adjusting the voltage supplied to the anode circuit, as described above. The method has the disadvantage that it does not allow fine regulation of the current. The selector switch

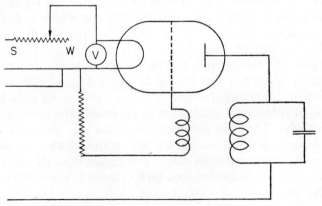

FIG. 141.—CONTROL OF CURRENT BY FILAMENT HEATING.

moves over studs and makes available several different voltages, but does not permit variations between these points.

THE FILAMENT HEATING. The intensity of the current passing across the valve, and so in the anode circuit, can be controlled by adjusting the heating of the filament of the valve. A series rheostat is included in the filament heating circuit (Fig. 141) and when all the resistance is in the circuit the intensity of the current passing through the filament is low; the filament does not become very hot, few electrons are emitted and the intensity of the current across the valve is small. As the resistance is reduced the intensity of current in the filament increases. This increases the heating of the filament, and so the emission of electrons, and the intensity of the current across the valve rises. A voltmeter is wired in parallel to the filament and shows the P.D. across it. This method permits fine regulation of the output, but is not widely used in modern machines, as the filament of the valve has a longer life if it operates at a constant temperature.

THE GRID BIAS. A charge applied to the grid influences the intensity of the current which flows across the valve, the more negative the grid, the less being the intensity of the current. The grid is connected to the filament by the grid leak circuit and a resistance is included in this circuit to maintain a difference of potential between the filament and the grid, the

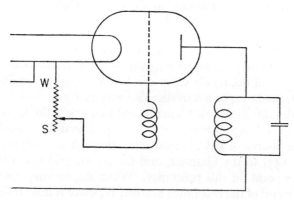

FIG. 142.—CONTROL OF CURRENT BY GRID BIAS.

former being the more negative. The P.D. between the filament and the grid varies directly with the value of this resistance, and when the control of current is by the grid bias a variable resistance is used (Fig. 142). Inclusion of a small part of the resistance results in a small P.D. between the filament and the grid, so the latter has a considerable negative bias and the intensity of the current flowing across the valve is low. As more resistance is included between the filament and the grid, the

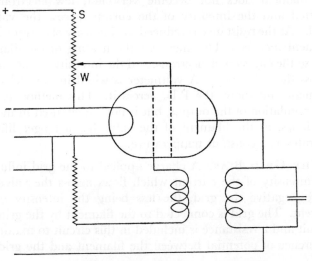

FIG. 143.—CONTROL OF CURRENT BY GRID BIAS
USING A TETRODE VALVE.

P.D. between them increases, the grid becomes less negative and the intensity of the current across the valve increases.

The grid of the triode valve can be employed to regulate the current, as above, or a tetrode valve may be used. This has four electrodes, an anode, a filament and two grids, the second, or screen grid lying between the first grid and the anode. A separate source of D.C. is connected through a resistance (WS in Fig. 143) to the filament, and the screen grid taken from a variable point on this resistance. When the moving contact is near the end of the resistance marked W, there is little resistance between the filament and the grid and so the P.D. between them is small. Consequently the grid has a negative bias and the intensity of the current across the valve is low. As the contact is moved towards S the resistance, and therefore the P.D., between the filament and the grid increases and the grid becomes less negative. This increases the intensity of the current that flows across the valve. Control of current by the grid bias has the advantages that fine regulation is obtained, while the filament is kept at a constant temperature.

COUPLING OF THE RESONATOR AND OSCILLATOR COILS. The relative position of the oscillator and resonator coils affects the intensity of the current that is induced in the latter, and in some machines the output is regulated by adjusting the position of the resonator coil.

TUNING OF THE RESONATOR AND OSCILLATOR CIRCUITS. This affects the output of the machine, but should not be used as a method of current regulation, as the machine operates most satisfactorily when the circuits are perfectly tuned.

Interference

High-frequency generators may interfere with the action of other electrical equipment and it is essential that appropriate steps are taken to prevent this. Interference can occur in various circumstances:

ELECTRONIC DEVICES. The electrical disturbances set up by the short-wave diathermic current can interfere with the action of electronic devices such as hearing aids, which may be damaged, and cardiac pacemakers, whose altered action may have serious consequences. Some hearing aids are constructed so that they are not affected, but for other electronic devices there is at present no solution other than avoiding close proximity to short-wave diathermic equipment and to other strong sources of electrical energy, which may have similar effects.

RADIO RECEPTION. The short-wave diathermic current sets up wireless waves which are liable to cause interference with radio and television reception and also with radio com-

I

munication between aircraft, ambulances, taxis, etc. Three frequencies have been allocated to medical work, the most suitable one being that of 27,120,000 cycles per second, which corresponds to a wave-length of 11 metres. Provided that waves of these frequencies only are emitted, there is no interference. Interference is, however, liable to occur in two ways:

(1) Slight variations in the frequency of the current produced by the machine. This can occur as a result of different arrangements of the electrodes and patient, which affect the capacity and inductance of the output circuit, or from slight variations within the machine. When using the frequency of 27,120,000 cycles per second variations between 27,000,000 and 27,240,000 cycles per second are permitted, but with the other two frequencies allocated to medial work less variation is allowed, and so these are rarely used.

(2) Production of harmonics. A circuit designed to produce a current of a certain frequency also generates currents of frequencies which are multiples of this fundamental frequency, *i.e.* harmonics. These set up wireless waves of shorter wavelength than those produced by the original current. The harmonics of 27,120,000 are 54,240,000, 81,360,000, etc.

Thus in eliminating interference with radio reception there are two problems to consider. One is the construction of a generator which operates only at the allocated frequency, and the other is the elimination of harmonics.

Various *frequency-stable generators* are available. One method of ensuring the production of a current of constant frequency is the inclusion of a quartz crystal in the circuit. If a potential difference is applied across such a crystal it causes distortion of the crystal, and conversely, if a crystal is distorted a potential difference is set up across it. The latter is termed the piezoelectric, the former the reverse piezoelectric effect, and once the crystal has been distorted a series of changes in shape tends to take place, *i.e.* the crystal oscillates, setting up a varying P.D. as it does so. The frequency of these oscillations depends on the way in which the crystal is cut, and is a constant factor for any particular crystal.

If a crystal is included in a circuit to which a high-frequency current is applied, the current can flow only if the crystal is in resonance with the current, *i.e.* if the two tend to oscillate with the same frequency. If this is not so the P.D. set up across the crystal stops the current flow. Inclusion of a crystal in the circuit gives a very stable frequency but for technical reasons the method is not completely satisfactory for a short-wave diathermic machine.

A more satisfactory method of ensuring that the current is of constant frequency is to replace the conventional coil and condenser circuit with another type of oscillator, such as the co-axial line or pot oscillator. These operate at a relatively stable frequency and are nowadays frequently used for the production of the short-wave diathermic current.

The other problem is the *elimination of harmonics* and although the oscillators mentioned above generate currents of a practically constant frequency, they also produce their harmonics. Consequently wireless waves of these different frequencies are liable to be emitted from both the oscillator circuit and the patient's circuit.

Emission from the oscillator circuit can be prevented by screening the circuit with a metal case, which prevents the passage of the waves. For effective screening of the coil and condenser oscillator, as used in the crystal circuit, a double screen is necessary. The pot and coaxial line oscillators require less screening, as each comprises a metal cylinder which acts as one screen, absorbing many of the waves. The metal case of the machine can form the second screen.

Screening of the oscillator does not prevent the transmission of harmonics to the output circuit, and emission of wireless waves of these frequencies from the electrode leads. This can, however, be prevented by including a "harmonic trap" in the resonator circuit. This is a device, consisting of choke coils and condensers, which allows the passage of a current of the fundamental frequency, but not of its harmonics. It works on the same principle as the mains filter used with the screening cubicle, which is described below.

OTHER ELECTRICAL EQUIPMENT. Short-wave diathermy may cause interference with other electrical equipment, such as the electrocardiograph. This is due in part to the electrical and magnetic disturbances set up but is also liable to occur when there are appreciable variations in the intensity of the current supplied to the high-frequency generator, as when an A.C. supply is used, and is due to sudden bursts of energy applied to the valve. Therefore the current supplied to the anode circuit of modern machines is commonly D.C., the A.C. of the supply being rectified by means of valves and smoothed by a condenser (Chapter 7). It is, however, a considerable advantage to screen any apparatus which is particularly susceptible to interference.

SCREENING CUBICLE. This was originally used to prevent interference with radio communications by short-wave diathermy. The patient and machine were enclosed in a special cubicle which absorbed the wireless waves set up by the short-wave diathermic current, so preventing their emission. A similar cubicle may be used to prevent outside electrical disturbances from reaching sensitive equipment such as the electrocardiograph and electromyograph, and interfering with their action. The floor, roof, and walls are made of sheets of metal or fine-mesh wire netting and are connected to earth. The metal absorbs the wireless waves, but to prevent their emission or entry the screening must be complete, with no conductors passing through it. If a conductor, such as a water pipe, passes through the screening, high-frequency currents may be induced in it within the screening, then flow along the conductor and set up wireless waves outside, or vice versa. The cables carrying the current to supply the machine must pass through the screening, and the passage of high-frequency currents along these cables is prevented by the use of a mains filter. This is connected to the cables at the point where they pass through the screening and consists of two choke coils, one on each lead, in series with the supply cables and two condensers in parallel to them (Fig. 144).

The choke coils offer considerable impedance to the high-frequency current, as inductive reactance to such a current is high, but the condensers offer little impedance as capacitive reactance is low. Therefore the high-frequency current takes the short circuit through the condensers instead of flowing along the main cables. The low-frequency current can pass

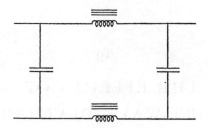

FIG. 144.—MAINS FILTER.

through the choke coils, but the high capacitive reactance prevents it from taking the short circuit through the condensers.

The principle of the harmonic trap is similar to the above, the condensers and choke coils being selected to allow the passage of the current of the fundamental frequency but not of its harmonics, of which the frequencies are higher.

19

THE EFFECTS OF
SHORT-WAVE DIATHERMY

THE short-wave diathermic current is a high-frequency alternating current which usually has a frequency of 27,120,000 cycles per second and sets up wireless waves with a wave-length of 11 metres. A high-frequency current does not stimulate motor or sensory nerves. When studying the muscle stimulating currents (Chapter 13) it was observed that, except with impulses of long duration, the shorter the duration of the impulse, the less was the effect on the nerves, 0·01 millisecond being the shortest duration of impulse generally used. A high-frequency current has a frequency of more than approximately 500,000 cycles per second. This provides 1,000,000 impulses per second, so each has a duration of 0·001 millisecond, which is beyond the range used for nerve stimulation. Thus when such a current is passed through the body there is no discomfort and no muscle contractions are produced. The current is evenly alternating, therefore there is no danger of chemical burns. Consequently it is possible to pass through the tissues currents of a much greater intensity than can be used with the direct and low-frequency currents. The intensity of the current can be great enough to produce a direct heating effect on the tissues, similar to the heating effect of the current on any other conductor, and the term diathermy means "through heating".

The frequency of the short-wave diathermic current is very high, so inductive reactance is considerable but capacitive reactance is fairly low. These properties make it possible to apply the short-wave diathermic current to the tissues by methods which cannot be used for other currents. There are two methods of application, the condenser field and cable methods.

The Condenser Field Method

PRINCIPLES. Electrodes are placed on each side of the part to be treated and separated from the skin by insulating material. The electrodes act as the plates of a condenser while the patient's tissues, together with the insulating material which separates them from the electrodes, form the dielectric. When the current is applied rapidly alternating charges are set up on the electrodes and give rise to a rapidly alternating electric field between them. The electric field influences the materials which lie within it.

EFFECTS OF THE ELECTRIC FIELD. A conductor is a material in which electrons can easily be displaced from their atoms, and when such a material lies within a varying electric

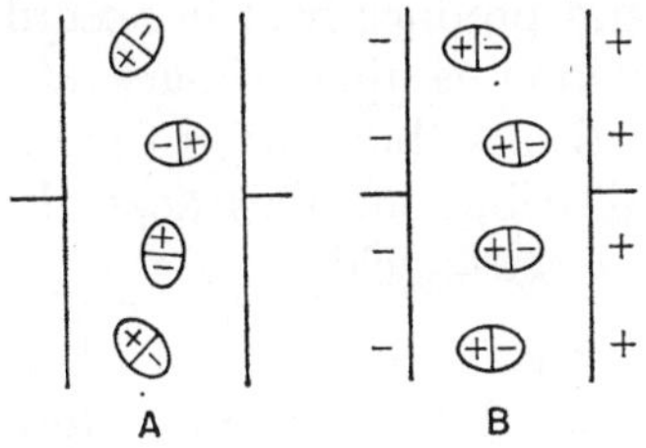

FIG. 145.—ROTATION OF DIPOLES.
A, condenser uncharged; B, condenser charged.

field there is a rapid oscillation of electrons and a high-frequency current is set up.

An electrolyte is a substance which contains ions, and when a varying electric field passes through an electrolyte the ions tend to move first in one direction then in the other. As the frequency of the short-wave diathermic current is very high, the result is vibration rather than actual movement of the ions. Electrolytes also contain dipoles, which are molecules consisting of two oppositely charged ions. The particle as a whole is electrically neutral, but one end bears a negative and the other a positive charge. As the electric field changes in direction the dipoles swing round so that each end lies as far as possible from the electrode bearing the same charge (Fig. 145). Thus in the electrolytes there is rotation of dipoles as well as vibration of ions.

An insulator is a substance in which the electrons are so firmly held by the central nuclei that they are not easily displaced from their atoms, and in such a substance the varying electric field causes molecular distortion. As the charges on the electrodes alternate and the molecules are distorted, the electron orbits swing first to one side, then to the other, and displacement currents are set up (Fig. 51, page 78).

In the body the tissue fluids are electrolytes, and when tissues containing an appreciable quantity of fluid lie in the electric field, vibration of ions and rotation of dipoles take place within them. Other tissues, such as fat, are virtually insulators and the effect of the electric field on these tissues is to produce molecular distortion. All these processes constitute electric currents and produce heat in accordance with Joule's law. Heat production is the primary effect of short-wave diathermy on the tissues, but differs from that of other heat treatments in its distribution. This depends primarily on the distribution of the electric field.

HEATING OF THE TISSUES. The characteristics of electric lines of force and their distribution form the basis of the following principles, and are considered fully in Chapters 1 and 6.

The electric field tends to spread between the electrodes and so its density is usually greatest close to the electrodes, be-

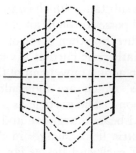

FIG. 146.—SPREAD OF LINES OF FORCE IN THE TISSUES.

coming less as the distance from them increases. The superficial tissues lie closer to the electrodes than do the deep ones,
so the density of the field, and consequently the heating, is
commonly greater in the superficial than in the deep tissues.
The lines of force pass more easily through materials of high
than of low dielectric constant, and as the tissues of the body
have a mean dielectric constant of about 80 they have a considerable effect on the distribution of the electric field. The
lines of force can travel easily through the tissues, so they tend
to spread considerably as they pass through the body (Fig. 146)
and this increases the tendency for the heating to be greater in
the superficial than in the deep tissues. An exception occurs

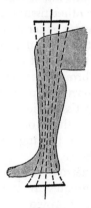

FIG. 147.—CONCENTRATION OF
LINES OF FORCE IN THE ANKLE.

when the cross-sectional area of the part is less than that of the
electrodes, as the lines of force travel through the tissues
rather than through the surrounding air. If, for example, one
electrode is placed on the sole of the foot and the other above
the flexed knee, the field density, and so the heating, is greatest
in the ankle (Fig. 147).

The dielectric constants of the various tissues differ considerably, those of low impedance, such as blood and muscle,
having much higher dielectric constants than the tissues with
a high impedance, such as fat and white fibrous tissue. The
relative arrangement of the tissues in the pathway of the electric

field affects the distribution of the lines of force, and so the heating. If the different tissues lie in parallel with each other the density of the field, and consequently the heat production, is greatest in the tissues of low impedance. This occurs when the field is passed longitudinally through a limb, when the blood, having the lowest impedance, is heated most. If, on the other hand, the tissues are in series with each other in the pathway of the electric field, the density of the lines of force is the same throughout and the tissues with the highest impedance are heated most. This corresponds to the heating of resistances which are wired in series with each other, as under these circumstances most heat is produced in the highest resistance. The subcutaneous tissue contains fat, which has a high impedance, and lies in series with the other tissues, so it is probable that an appreciable amount of heat is generated in this region. Usually the arrangement of the tissues is such that they do not offer a true series or parallel pathway but a mixture of the two. The lines of force must pass through the skin, superficial fascia and muscle, but then have alternative pathways through the underlying tissues. As the deep tissues lie in parallel with each other, the heating is greatest in those of low impedance and it is difficult to obtain a direct heating effect on deeply placed structures of high impedance.

When short-wave diathermy is applied to the body the heat production tends to be greatest in the superficial tissues and those of low impedance, but provided that a suitable method of application is chosen the treatment provides as deep a form of heat as any available to the physiotherapist. In addition there is some rise in temperature in tissues which are not heated directly by the current. Tissues in contact with those in which the heat is produced are heated by conduction of heat, so when the muscles surrounding a deeply placed joint are heated some heat is transmitted to the joint. As the blood circulates through the area in which the heat is produced its temperature rises and heat is carried to adjacent tissues through which it passes.

HEAT LOSS. The blood passing through the part that is being treated carries heat away from this area. This occurs particularly in vascular areas, and as the temperature of the part rises the blood vessels dilate and the effect is increased.

For this reason all forms of heat should be applied gradually, to allow for vasodilatation to take place and heat loss to be established. If any factor impedes the flow of blood through the area the heat is not carried away and overheating is liable to occur. Heat is also lost by conduction to surrounding tissues and to some extent by radiation and the evaporation of sweat from the surface.

The Cable Method

PRINCIPLES. The electrode consists of a thick, insulated cable which completes the patient's circuit of the machine. The cable is coiled in relationship to the patient's tissues, but separated from them by a layer of insulating material. As the high-frequency current oscillates in the cable an electrostatic field is set up between its ends (the antinodes of potential) and a

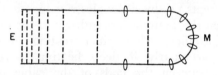

FIG. 148.—ELECTRIC AND MAGNETIC FIELDS AROUND THE CABLE ELECTRODE.
E = electric field   M = magnetic field

magnetic field around its centre (the node of potential). These fields are shown in Fig. 148 and affect the tissues that lie within them.

THE ELECTROSTATIC FIELD. The tissues which lie between the ends of the cable are in the electrostatic field, and the effects on these tissues are similar to those produced when the current is applied by the condenser field method. The distribution of the field follows the same principles, so while the heating tends to be greatest in the superficial tissues and those of low impedance it should be possible, provided that suitable technique is used, to obtain some heating of the more deeply placed structures of high impedance.

THE MAGNETIC FIELD. The magnetic field varies as the current oscillates and EMFs are produced by electromagnetic induction in any conductor which is cut by the magnetic lines of force. If the conductor is a solid piece of conducting material the EMFs give rise to eddy currents (Chapter 5), and these currents are produced in the tissues which lie close to the centre of the cable. The eddy currents produce heat, and as they are set up only in conductors the effect is confined to the tissues of low impedance and heating of the subcutaneous fat is avoided. The currents are produced primarily near the surface of the conductor, so it is the superficial tissues that are affected most. As with the other methods, some heat is transferred to adjacent tissues by conduction and by the circulation of the heated blood, but the effects are primarily on the superficial tissues of low impedance.

RELATIVE EFFECTS OF THE TWO FIELDS. It has been shown experimentally that if the cable is coiled round material of high impedance the electric field predominates, while the currents produced by electromagnetic induction are strongest when the material around which the cable is coiled is of low impedance. Thus when treating an area of high impedance, particularly if deep heating is required, the electric field between the ends of the cable is utilised in preference to the magnetic field at its centre. In this case the electric field predominates over the magnetic field, and also it is more effective than the magnetic field for heating the deeply placed structures and those of high impedance. When treating an area of low impedance, particularly if superficial heating is required, the eddy currents set up by the magnetic field at the centre of the cable are utilised in preference to the electric field. In tissues of low impedance these currents predominate over the electric field, and they produce a satisfactory heating of the superficial structures. Both effects can be utilised at the same time. If the whole cable is arranged in relationship to the patient's tissues, an electric field is set up between its ends, and eddy currents near its centre.

Physiological Effects

The principal effect of the short-wave diathermic current on the body is the production of heat in the tissues, and the physiological effects result from the rise of temperature.

INCREASED METABOLISM. Van't Hoff's law states that any chemical change capable of being accelerated by heat is accelerated by rise of temperature. Consequently heating of the tissues accelerates the chemical changes, *i.e.* the metabolism. Oxygen and foodstuffs are used up, so that there is an increased demand for them, and the output of waste products is increased.

INCREASED BLOOD SUPPLY. As a result of the increased metabolism the output of waste products from the cells is increased. These include metabolites, which act on the walls of the capillaries and arterioles, causing dilatation of these vessels. In addition the heat has a direct effect on the blood vessels, causing vasodilatation, particularly in the superficial tissues where the heating is greatest. Stimulation of superficial sensory nerve endings can cause a reflex dilatation of the arterioles, but this effect is probably less important with short-wave diathermy than with methods of heating which cause a more marked irritation of the sensory nerve endings in the skin. As a result of the vasodilatation there is an increased flow of blood through the area, so that the necessary oxygen and nutritive materials are supplied, and waste products are removed.

EFFECT ON NERVES. Provided that the heating is not excessive, it appears to reduce the excitability of nerves.

EFFECTS ON MUSCLE TISSUE. Rise in temperature induces relaxation of muscles and increases the efficiency of their action. The muscle fibres contract and relax more quickly, although the strength of the contraction is not affected, and relaxation of the antagonists permits a freer action of the prime movers. The increased blood supply ensures the optimum conditions for muscle contraction.

DESTRUCTION OF TISSUES. Excessive heating causes coagulation, and so destruction of the tissues.

GENERAL RISE IN TEMPERATURE. As blood passes through the tissues in which the rise of temperature has occurred, it also becomes heated and carries the heat to other parts of the body. Thus if the heating is fairly extensive and prolonged a general rise in the body temperature occurs. The vasomotor centre is affected and a generalised dilatation of superficial blood-vessels results.

FALL IN BLOOD PRESSURE. The generalised vasodilatation mentioned above reduces the peripheral resistance to the blood flow. The heat also causes a reduction in the viscosity of the blood and these two factors together result in a fall in blood pressure.

INCREASED ACTIVITY OF SWEAT GLANDS. If a general rise of temperature occurs there tends to be increased activity of the sweat glands throughout the body. In addition, local heating of the skin increases the activity of the glands in the affected area, although this effect should not be very great with short-wave diathermy as strong heating of the skin is avoided.

Therapeutic Effects and Uses

EFFECTS ON INFLAMMATORY PROCESSES. The dilatation of arterioles and capillaries results in an increased flow of blood to the area, making available an increased supply of oxygen and nutritive materials, and also bringing more antibodies and white blood cells. The dilatation of capillaries increases the exudation of fluid into the tissues and this is followed by increased absorption which, together with the increased flow of blood through the area, assists in the removal of waste products. These effects help to bring about the resolution of inflammation. The additional effects obtained when the inflammation is associated with bacterial infection are considered below.

In the acute stages of inflammation caution should be exercised in applying the treatment to areas in which there is already marked vasodilatation and exudation of fluid, as an increase in these processes may aggravate the symptoms. In the subacute stages stronger doses may be applied, with considerable benefit. When the inflammation is chronic a thermal dose of fairly long duration must be used to be effective. Short-wave diathermy is particularly valuable for lesions of deeply placed structures, such as the hip joint, which cannot easily be affected by other forms of electrotherapy and radiations. The above effects are of value, in conjunction with other forms of physiotherapy, in various inflammatory conditions, *e.g.* rheumatoid arthritis, capsulitis, tendinitis, and for the inflammatory changes which frequently occur in the ligaments surrounding osteo-arthritic joints.

EFFECTS IN BACTERIAL INFECTIONS. Inflammation is the normal response of the tissues to the presence of bacteria, the principal features being vasodilatation, exudation of fluid into the tissues and increase in the white blood cells and antibodies in the area. The response obtained on heating the tissues augments these changes and so reinforces the body's normal mechanism for dealing with the infecting organisms. Therefore short-wave diathermy is frequently of value in the treatment of bacterial infections such as boils, carbuncles and abscesses. Treatment in the early stages may occasionally bring about resolution of the inflammation without pus formation occurring, but failing this the changes are accelerated. Until there is free drainage the treatment should be given cautiously, as for all cases of acute inflammation. When the abscess is draining freely stronger doses may be applied, the increased blood supply assisting the healing processes once the infection has been overcome.

In some cases short-wave diathermy appears to aggravate the condition, but increased discharge for a few days is an indication of acceleration of the changes occurring in the tissues, and not a contraindication to treatment. Should the increased discharge persist, it may be an indication that the body's defence mechanism is already taxed to its uttermost, so that it is impossible to reinforce its action. This is most liable to occur in cases of longstanding infection, and under these circumstances no benefit is derived from the application of short-wave diathermy.

Bacteria can be destroyed directly by heat, but it would be impossible to raise the body tissues to the necessary temperature without causing damage to the tissues themselves.

EFFECTS IN TRAUMATIC CONDITIONS. The beneficial effects on traumatic lesions are similar to those produced in inflammation. The exudation of fluid, followed by increased absorption, and the increased flow of blood through the area assist in the removal of waste products, while the improved blood supply makes available more nutritive materials, so assisting the healing processes.

Recent injuries should be treated with the same caution as acute inflammation, as excessive heating is liable to increase the exudation of fluid from the damaged vessels. Stiff joints and other after-effects of injury require stronger doses, the treatment being a preliminary to the exercise which is usually the essential part of the treatment.

EFFECTS IN CIRCULATORY DEFECTS.   As a result of the vasodilatation, there is increased blood supply to the tissues. This may be used in conditions where the circulation is poor and the limb cold, e.g. anterior poliomyelitis.

When the poor circulation is associated with defective arterial blood supply, heat should not be applied directly to the affected area. The increased metabolism increases the demand of the tissues for oxygen, but the arterial defect may make it impossible to achieve the increase in blood flow necessary to supply this. In such cases gangrene of the tissues may be precipitated by the local application of heat. An indirect method of increasing the blood supply may, however, be used. If diathermy is applied through the abdomen for an adequate length of time, dilatation of the peripheral vessels takes place. This is probably due to heating of the blood, which affects the vasomotor centre and causes generalised dilatation of the superficial blood vessels. There is some doubt as to the value of this treatment, as the vasodilatation can only be maintained for short periods, i.e. during and immediately after the treatment.

RELIEF OF PAIN.   It is found that a mild degree of heating is effective in relieving pain, presumably as a result of a sedative effect on the sensory nerves. It is thought that pain may be due to the accumulation in the tissues of the "P" substance, a waste product of metabolism, and that the increased flow of blood through the area assists in removing this substance, so relieving pain. Strong superficial heating probably relieves pain by counter-irritation, but it is unlikely that the heating of the skin produced by short-wave diathermy is great enough to have this effect. When pain is due to inflammatory processes, resolution of the inflammation is accompanied by relief of pain. Short-wave diathermy assists in bringing about the resolution of inflammation, and so indirectly in relieving the pain. Strong heating may, however, cause an increase of pain, especially in acute inflammation, if the increased blood flow and exudation of fluid cause an increase of tension in the tissues.

Thus, when short-wave diathermy is used in the treatment of inflammatory and post-traumatic lesions, it brings about relief of pain in addition to the effects mentioned previously. This is particularly valuable when the treatment forms a preliminary to active exercise, which can subsequently be performed more efficiently.

EFFECTS ON MUSCLE TISSUE. The heating of the tissues induces muscle relaxation, and so short-wave diathermy may be used for the relief of muscle spasm associated with inflammation and trauma, usually as a preliminary to movements. Increased efficiency of muscle action should also aid the satisfactory performance of active exercises.

The treatment has been used in an attempt to reduce muscle spasm due to upper motor neurone lesions, but other methods of inducing relaxation are more satisfactory for these cases.

GENERAL RISE IN TEMPERATURE AND FALL IN BLOOD PRESSURE. In the past these effects have been utilised for the treatment of subnormal temperature and high blood pressure, but they are too transient to have any value.

20

THE APPLICATION OF SHORT-WAVE DIATHERMY

The Condenser Field Method

WHEN short-wave diathermy is applied by the condenser field method, the heat production is determined by the distribution of the electric field and tends to be greatest in the superficial tissues and those of low impedance. The tendency for the heating to be confined to these areas can be minimised by suitable arrangement of the electrodes. In order to obtain deep heating it is necessary to avoid overheating the skin, as the resulting sensation of warmth limits the current tolerated. In most cases the aim is to achieve as even a field as possible in the deep and superficial tissues.

SIZE OF ELECTRODES. As a general rule the electrodes should be rather larger than the structure that is being treated. The electric field tends to spread, particularly at the edges, resulting in a lower density, and so less heating, in the deep

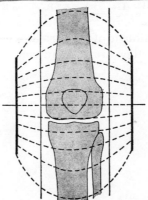

FIG. 149.—JOINT LYING IN CENTRAL, EVEN PART OF ELECTRIC FIELD.

than in the superficial tissues. If the electrodes are large the outer part of the field, where the spread is greatest, is deliberately not utilised, the structure lying in the more even, central part of the field (Fig. 149). For treatments of the trunk the electrodes should be as large as possible, while for a limb they should be rather larger than the diameter of the limb.

The tissues of the body have a higher dielectric constant than air. Consequently, if the part of a limb between the electrodes is smaller in diameter than the electrodes, the lines of force bend in towards the limb (Fig. 150). If the diameter of the

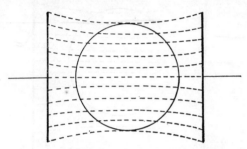

FIG. 150.—CORRECT SIZE OF ELECTRODES.

electrodes is smaller than that of the limb, the lines of force spread in the tissues, causing more heating of the superficial than of the deep structures (Fig. 151). If the diameter of the electrodes is far larger than that of the limb, some of the lines of force pass each side through the air and part of the electrical energy is wasted, though a satisfactory heating effect is obtained (Fig. 152).

Large electrodes allow the use of wider spacing than is

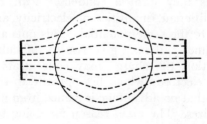

FIG. 151.—ELECTRODES TOO SMALL.

possible with small ones, and wide spacing has certain advantages, which are considered in the next section. The condenser formed by the electrodes and intervening materials impedes the flow of current, on account of the capacitive reactance, and the smaller the capacity of the condenser, the greater is the capacitive reactance. The capacity of the condenser varies directly with the size of the plates and inversely with the width

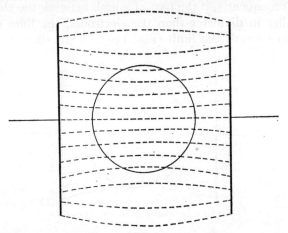

FIG. 152.—ELECTRODES TOO LARGE.

of the dielectric. So with large electrodes wide spacing can be used without forming a condenser with unduly small capacity, which would cause excessive impedance. Wide spacing with small electrodes forms a condenser with a very small capacity, and gives rise to considerable capacitive reactance.

Both electrodes should be of the same size. If they are of different sizes they form a condenser with different sized plates, and different quantities of electricity are required to charge them to the same potential. This puts an uneven load on the machine, and may give rise to difficulties in tuning. Apart from this, the charge may concentrate on that part of the larger electrode which lies opposite to the smaller one (Fig. 153) so that no advantage is gained from using electrodes of different sizes. The main reason for doing so would be to obtain different degrees of heating under the two electrodes, and this can be achieved more satisfactorily by adjusting the spacing.

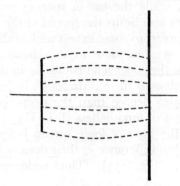

FIG. 153.—ELECTRODES OF DIFFERENT SIZES.

ELECTRODE SPACING. The spacing between the electrodes and the patient's tissues should be as wide as the output of the machine allows, and the material between the electrodes and the skin should be of low dielectric constant, air being the most satisfactory.

The lines of force spread as they pass between the plates of a charged condenser, particularly if the distance between the plates is small and the material between them of high dielectric

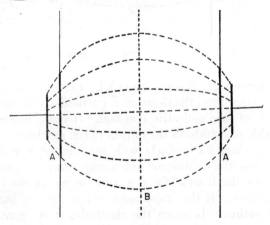

FIG. 154.—ELECTRODES CLOSE TO SURFACES.

constant. When the electrode spacing is wide the distance between the electrodes is large so the spread of the electric field is minimal, while the use of spacing material of a low dielectric constant also limits the spread of the field. The field does, however, spread to some extent and so the density of the lines of force is greatest close to the electrodes. When the spacing is narrow the superficial tissues lie in the concentrated part of the field close to the electrodes (A in Fig. 154) and are heated to a greater degree than the deep tissues where the density of the lines of force is less (B in Fig. 154). When the spacing is wide the lines of force spread before reaching the skin and there is less difference in their density in the deep and superficial tissues (Fig. 155). Thus wide spacing helps to

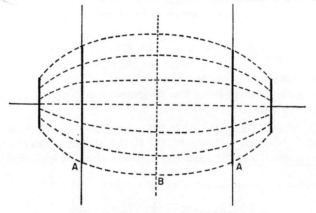

FIG. 155.—ELECTRODES FURTHER FROM SURFACES.

reduce the tendency for the superficial tissues to be heated to a greater extent than the deep ones, particularly if the spacing material is of low dielectric constant. It does, however, put considerable demands on the output of the machine.

Wide spacing, particularly with material of low dielectric constant, has the additional advantage that it reduces the tendency for the lines of force to concentrate in the tissues of low impedance. If the impedance of the spacing material is high the pathway between the electrodes offers considerable impedance to the lines of force. The different tissues offer different impedances, but where the total impedance of the pathway is great, these slight variations have little effect on the whole, so the distribution of the field is relatively even.

If one electrode is placed nearer to the skin than the other there is a greater sensation of heat under the nearer electrode than under the further one. This is illustrated in Fig. 156. The

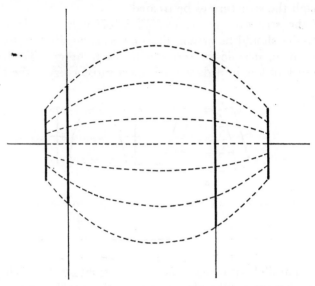

FIG. 156.—ELECTRODES AT UNEQUAL DISTANCES FROM SURFACES.

lines of force under the further electrode have a greater distance in which to spread before reaching the skin than those under the nearer one. They therefore cover a greater area of skin and their density is less under the further than under the nearer electrode. When treating a structure which lies nearer to one surface of the body than to the other, e.g. the hip joint, the directing electrode on the further surface is placed at a greater distance from the skin than the active. This reduces the possibility of the patient experiencing a greater sensation of heat under the directing electrode than under the active, which, if it did occur, might limit the total current tolerated. The principle is the same as that underlying the use of a large directing electrode when applying the direct or low frequency currents, but with short-wave diathermy different degrees of heating are obtained more satisfactorily by using different spacing than by using different sized electrodes.

POSITION OF ELECTRODES. The position of the electrodes should be chosen with the aim of directing the electric field through the structure to be treated.

If the structure to be treated is of high impedance the electrodes should be arranged, as far as is possible, so that the different tissues lie in series with each other. To heat a structure of low impedance it is most satisfactory if the tissues

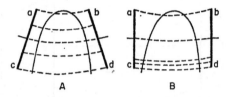

A   B

FIG. 157.—POSITION OF ELECTRODES RELATIVE TO THE SURFACE OF THE BODY.
A. Correct.   B. Incorrect.

are in parallel with each other. When treating the ankle joint electrodes are commonly placed on the medial and lateral aspects, the tissues lie in series with each other and some heating of the joint should be obtained. If a longitudinal application is used a sensation of warmth is experienced in the ankle region, but as the tissues lie in parallel with each other the heating is mainly confined to the blood vessels and muscles. The latter method would be satisfactory for treatment of the soft structures.

The electrodes should be placed parallel to the skin, otherwise the field concentrates on the area of tissue lying closest to the electrode. The insulating material between the electrodes and the skin has a low dielectric constant, so offers considerable impedance to the lines of force, the majority of which take the shortest pathway through it. Placing the electrodes parallel to the skin may result in their not lying parallel to each other, but, provided that the extra length of pathway between the more widely separate parts of the electrodes is through the body tissues, this has little effect on the field distribution. The tissues have a high dielectric constant, so the lines of force can travel through them easily, and the longer pathway offers little more impedance than the shorter one. Fig. 157 represents the lateral aspect of the shoulder, which is narrower above than below. If the electrodes lie parallel to the skin they are at a slight angle to each other, but an even field is obtained (Fig. 157A). The pathway *cd* is longer than *ab*, but the extra length is through the body tissues and the two pathways have about the same impedance. If, however, the electrodes are placed vertically (Fig. 157B), the field tends to concentrate between their lower parts. The pathways *ab* and *cd* are of the same length, but much more of *ab* than of *cd* is through the air. Consequently *ab* has the greater impedance and the field tends to concentrate between *c* and *d*.

Care must be taken that the distance between the electrodes is greater than the total width of spacing. In Fig. 158 the

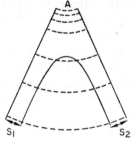

FIG. 158.—ELECTRODES TOO CLOSE TO EACH OTHER.

distance between the electrodes at A is less than the total spacing (s_1+s_2) and many of the lines of force pass directly from one electrode to the other, not through the tissues.

Electrodes should, where possible, be placed over an even surface of the body. Should the surface be irregular, the field tends to concentrate on the more prominent parts (Fig. 159A). Where an irregular surface cannot be avoided, the concentration can be reduced by using wide spacing. In Fig. 159A, the distance between the electrodes and the skin at *a* is less than half that at *b*, and so the field concentrates at *a*. In Fig. 159B there is much less difference in the distance between the skin and electrode at *a* and at *b*, and the field is much more even.

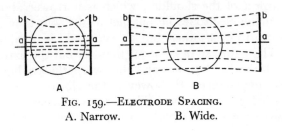

FIG. 159.—ELECTRODE SPACING.
A. Narrow.   B. Wide.

Various methods of arranging the electrodes may be used:

(1) *Contraplanar.* This method is usually the most satisfactory, especially for the treatment of deeply placed structures. The electrodes are placed over opposite aspects of the trunk or limb, so that the electric field is directed through the deep tissues. If the structure is nearer to one surface of the body than to the other the directing electrode, on the more distant surface, is placed further away from the skin than the active. The position of the electrodes can, if necessary, be modified, so that they do not lie exactly opposite to each other. Provided that they are both parallel to the skin, and do not approach too close to each other, a satisfactory field can be obtained.

(2) *Coplanar.* Electrodes can be placed side by side on the same aspect of the part, provided that there is an adequate distance between them. The pathway through the tissues offers less impedance to the lines of force than that through the air

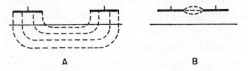

FIG. 160.—COPLANAR ARRANGEMENT OF ELECTRODES.
A. Correct.   B. Incorrect.

between the electrodes, so the distribution of the field is as shown in Fig. 160A. It is important that the distance between the electrodes is more than the total width of spacing, otherwise the electric field will not pass through the tissues (Fig. 160B). The heating is more superficial than with the contraplanar method, but is satisfactory for certain areas. Superficial structures which are too extensive for a contraplanar application may be treated in this way, as, for example, the spine, which can be heated with electrodes over the dorsal and lumbar regions.

The method is particularly suitable for the treatment of superficial structures where some factor contraindicates the placing of an electrode immediately over the lesion. When a boil is treated the prominence tends to cause concentration of the field on the apex of the boil, and as pus has a high dielectric constant it also tends to cause concentration of the field. In addition there may be loss of cutaneous sensation, which makes it unsafe to place an electrode immediately over the area. For such a case the coplanar method would be the most suitable. It is also of value for treating superficial lesions when heating of the deep structures is undesirable, e.g. a stitch abscess following an abdominal operation.

(3) *Cross-Fire Treatment.* Half the treatment is given with the electrodes in one position, then the arrangement is changed so that the electric field lies at right angles to that obtained during the first part of the treatment, e.g. for the knee joint, half the treatment would be given with the electrodes over the

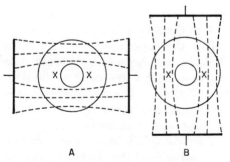

A   B

Fig. 161.—Cross-Fire Treatment.

medial and lateral aspects, the other half with them over the anterior and posterior aspects.

This method is used to treat the walls of cavities containing air, *e.g.* the frontal or maxillary sinuses, or the lungs. The lines of force pass through the tissues between the electrodes, but avoid the cavity, as the air within it has a low dielectric constant. Thus those walls of the cavity which face the electrodes are not treated (XX in Fig. 161A). If the position of the electrodes is then changed, so that the field lies at right angles to the previous one, these walls are heated (Fig. 161B).

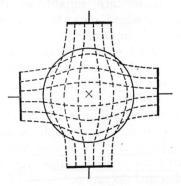

FIG. 162.—CROSS-FIRE TREATMENT.

The cross-fire method may also be used for the treatment of deeply placed structures, particularly if they lie in extensive vascular areas, *e.g.* the pelvic organs, the hip joint. The dielectric constant of the vascular tissues is very high, and the cross-sectional area of the part larger than the electrodes, so the field spreads in the deep tissues, which consequently receive less heating than the superficial ones. By passing the field through the area in two directions, the deep tissues (x in Fig. 162) receive twice as long a treatment as the skin.

(4) *Monopolar Technique.* The active electrode is placed over the site of the lesion and the other, indifferent electrode is applied to some distant part of the body, or may not be used at all. A separate electric field is set up under each electrode, the lines of force radiating from the electrode (Fig. 163). Thus the density of the field becomes less as the distance from the elec-

trode increases, and the heating is superficial. The method is
unsuitable for deeply placed structures, though it may be used
for very superficial lesions, *e.g.* treatment of the eye.

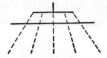

FIG. 163.—MONOPOLAR TECHNIQUE.

The Cable Method

When short-wave diathermy is applied by the cable method,
the effect of the electric field may be utilised, or that of the
magnetic field, or use may be made of both effects at the
same time.

The electric lines of force pass between the antinodes, and in
order to make full use of the electric field the ends of the cable
should lie as far as possible from each other, at the limits of
the application, so that the electric lines of force pass through
the whole of the area included (Fig. 164). The magnetic lines
of force are chiefly around the node and in order to obtain
maximum effect from the eddy currents that they produce the
centre of the cable is used, care being taken that the coil is

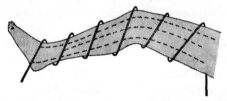

FIG. 164.—WHOLE CABLE APPLIED TO THE LOWER LIMB.

wound in the same direction throughout, otherwise opposing
magnetic fields are set up and energy lost.

For treatment of the limbs the cable is usually coiled round
the part. If the area is extensive, as when treating the whole
of a limb, or two limbs, all the cable is used and both electrostatic and magnetic fields are utilised. When treating a smaller
area the whole of the cable may not be required and either
the ends or the centre may be used, according to the depth of

heating required and the impedance of the tissues. If the area is of high impedance the electrostatic field between the ends of the cable is most effective. For the knee joint, two turns may be made with each end of the cable, these lying above and below the joint (Fig. 165). When treating two joints, *e.g.*

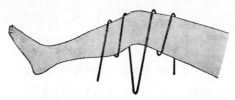

FIG. 165.—ENDS OF CABLE APPLIED TO THE KNEE.

both shoulders, a few turns may be made with one end of the cable round one joint and a similar arrangement of the other end round the other joint. If the area to be treated is of low impedance the eddy currents produce satisfactory heating, so

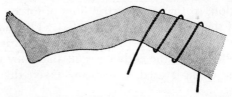

FIG. 166.—CENTRE OF CABLE APPLIED TO THE THIGH.

the centre of the cable is used, *e.g.* for muscles of the calf or thigh (Fig. 166).

To treat a flat surface, such as the back or abdomen, the cable can be arranged in a flat helix (Fig. 167), two helices made from its ends (Fig. 170), or a grid arrangement may be

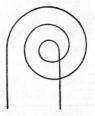

FIG. 167.—CABLE ARRANGED IN FLAT
SPIRAL.

used (Fig. 168). With the latter the magnetic field is complex and probably does not penetrate very deeply into the tissues, so heating is mainly by the electric field, but with the other two methods the tissues are heated by eddy currents. These flow at right angles to the magnetic lines of force and the heating produced by a single helix is in the form of a hollow

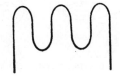

FIG. 168.—GRID ARRANGEMENT OF CABLE.

ring in the tissues lying under the coil. Fig. 169 illustrates this. In the left-hand diagram the coil is viewed from the side, the broken lines show the magnetic lines of force and the continuous line the eddy currents. In the right-hand diagram the coil is viewed from above and the shading shows the area in which heat is produced. When the double helix is used the magnetic

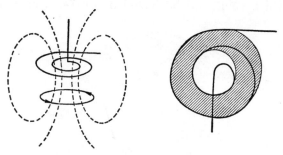

FIG. 169.—HEATING WITH A SINGLE HELIX.

lines of force link the two coils, as shown in Fig. 170. Eddy currents are produced in the tissues lying between the two helices, so heating is in this area, being greatest in the superficial tissues, where the eddy currents are closest together. Care must be taken that there is a reasonable distance between the two helices, otherwise intense heating could cause a burn. The two coils may be placed on a flat surface, as in Fig. 170, or they may be arranged on opposite aspects of the body, in a similar manner to condenser electrodes.

The cable may be used in conjunction with one condenser electrode, and the method is useful for the treatment of the

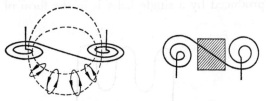

FIG. 170.—HEATING WITH A DOUBLE HELIX.

hip joint when flexion deformity renders an anteroposterior application of condenser electrodes unsuitable. The cable is coiled round the thigh, one end is attached to the machine and the other is insulated, often with a crutch rubber. A condenser electrode is placed level with the sacrum, but on the side of the affected hip, and directs the electric field through the region of the hip (Fig. 171).

The cable method is useful for the treatment of an extensive area, which could not be included between condenser elec-

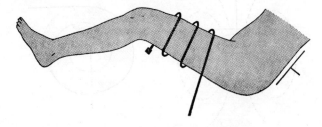

FIG. 171.—TREATMENT OF THE HIP JOINT.

trodes, also when the area is irregular, as with hands affected by rheumatoid arthritis, and when it is desirable to avoid heating the subcutaneous fat. Its disadvantage is the impossibility of using air spacing, so that the skin is liable to become warm and limit the effect that can be obtained on the deep tissues.

MONODE ELECTRODE. The monode works on the same principle as the cable. It consists of a flat helix of thick wire mounted in a rigid support. A condenser in parallel with the coil makes it possible to use a shorter length of wire than that required for the cable. Heating is produced by eddy currents and is in the form of a hollow ring, like that of the single helix, but the rigid support enables the electrode to be used with air spacing.

Technique of Application

TESTING OF THE MACHINE. The machine should be tested before use. When condenser electrodes are to be used these are arranged opposite to each other, with a gap between. The operator places her hand between the electrodes, switches on and tunes the machine, then increases the current until a comfortable warmth is felt. When the cable is to be used this may be arranged in a single loop and tested with a neon tube, which lights up opposite the antinodes when an adequate current is applied. Alternatively the cable can be coiled round the operator's arm and the current applied as before until warmth is felt. After testing, the controls are returned to zero.

PREPARATION OF THE PATIENT. The couch, chair or table that is used for supporting the patient should not contain metal, as this is liable to distort the electric field and to be heated by currents which may be induced in it. A deck chair is satisfactory as electrodes can be placed behind the canvas.

Clothing is removed from the area to be treated, which must be dry. If the area is damp the moisture on the surface of the skin is heated quickly and gives rise to a sensation of warmth, which limits the intensity of current that can be applied. Clothing may be slightly damp from perspiration, and its presence interferes with the circulation of air, which aids the evaporation of any sweat which may form during the treatment. It may, if tight, interfere with the flow of blood through the area, with consequent overheating, or, if the patient is resting on an electrode, it may cause uneven pressure. If the clothing is not removed, the necessary inspection of the skin before and after treatment is not possible, and the skin-electrode distance

K

and position of the electrodes cannot be judged accurately. The presence of clothing makes it difficult for the patient to appreciate the sensation of warmth, and metal objects may pass undetected. Metal and moisture both have a high dielectric constant, and a localised area of either causes concentration of an electric field, with consequent overheating. Metal objects, and anything that is damp, should be removed from the vicinity of the area to be treated, *i.e.* from within at least 1 foot of the electrodes. Wounds and sinuses must be cleansed and covered with a dry dressing before commencing treatment.

The patient must be comfortable and the part to be treated fully supported, as movement may alter the skin-electrode distance.

The ammeter is no guide to the amount of heating of the tissues, and is merely of value for tuning the circuits. Consequently the dose is estimated by the amount of heat felt by the patient. It is therefore very important for the patient to understand the degree of warmth that he should feel, that undue heat should be reported and that there is a danger of burns if the heat becomes excessive.

Skin sensation must be tested before the first treatment, and the test may be carried out with test tubes, one of which contains warm and the other cold water. Should the sensation be defective in any part of the area, it is unwise to apply the treatment. The vasomotor response in an insensitive area is less than that in a normal one, heat is not carried away so quickly and overheating is liable to occur.

Hearing aids must be removed and left well away from the machine, as induced currents may cause serious damage to them.

THE ELECTRODES. There are various types of condenser electrode, but each consists of a metal plate surrounded by some form of insulating material. One type has a glass cover, within which the position of the metal plate can be adjusted. These electrodes are commonly circular, but special shapes are made for some irregular areas, such as the axilla. Electrodes of this type are arranged in position on supporting arms and it is advisable to leave a small gap between the glass and the skin to allow for the circulation of air. Similar electrodes are made with a Bakelite or plastic cover instead of glass.

Another type of electrode consists of a rigid metal plate coated with a thin layer of insulating material, either rubber or plastic. The plates are frequently convex at the edges, and this type provides a more even electric field than a flat disc. An electric charge concentrates at the edges of a conductor and sets up a more intense electric field in this area than elsewhere. With the convex electrodes the edges are further from the skin than is the centre, so the peripheral part of the field has room to spread before reaching the skin, where the distribution is even (Fig. 172). These electrodes are arranged in position on supporting arms and are separated from the skin by an air gap.

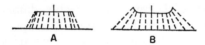

FIG. 172.—ELECTRIC FIELDS FROM:
A. FLAT; B. CONVEX ELECTRODES.

They may have an adjustable device projecting from the centre to ensure correct spacing.

A third type of electrode consists of a malleable metal plate covered with a thin layer of rubber. This can be moulded to the part, but should not be bent sharply or the metal plate may crack. Electrodes of this type are separated from the skin by perforated felt and may be fixed with a strap or bandage, or the body weight may be sufficient to maintain their position. The felt is perforated so that it contains a proportion of air, which is the most satisfactory spacing material, but the impossibility of using entirely air spacing is one of the disadvantages of this type of electrode.

The cable electrode consists of a thick wire covered with rubber. It is separated from the skin by at least four layers of dry turkish towelling, forming a thickness of half an inch or more. The turns of the cable should be at least one inch apart and may be secured with spacers made of insulating material.

POSITION AND SIZE OF ELECTRODES. This has been considered in the sections on the condenser field and cable methods of treatment. When arranging the electrodes it is important to remember that an electric field can be set up from the edges and back of the electrode as well as from the front. If these parts approach too close to the patient's tissues a field is set up in this area, and may cause uncomfortable heating, *e.g.* when treating one knee joint the back of the electrode placed on the medial aspect of the joint may lie too close to the other knee, which is consequently heated.

THE LEADS. In all cases the leads or cable must be of the correct length for the particular electrodes and machine that are used (Chapter 17). The leads should lie parallel to each other, at least as far apart as the terminals of the machine, and not approach close to any conductor. Currents may be induced in any conductor which lies near to the leads, with consequent loss of energy and possible damage from over-heating. Similarly the leads must be separated from the patient's skin by a distance at least as great as the electrode spacing, otherwise currents are induced in the tissues and cause heating in this area.

APPLICATION OF CURRENT. When the patient, electrodes, and leads are in position, the current is turned on and the circuits tuned. The current is then turned up slowly, allowing time for vasodilatation to occur and for the patient to appreciate the degree of heating. The operator should remain within call of the patient throughout the treatment, and turn the current off immediately if the heating becomes excessive.

At the end of the treatment the controls are returned to zero, the current switched off and the electrodes removed. The skin may be faintly pink, but there should be no strong reaction. Notes are kept of the size and spacing of the electrodes, the meter reading, the duration of the treatment and any reaction that is observed.

DOSAGE. In most cases the intensity of the application should be sufficient to cause a comfortable warmth and the duration of the treatment 20 to 30 minutes. For the treatment of chronic inflammatory lesions a duration of at least 30 minutes is desirable. The applications may be carried out daily, or on alternate days.

For the treatment of acute inflammation or recent injury the application should be less intense than that suggested above, but may be carried out more frequently, *e.g.* twice daily. The current may be sufficient to produce a mild sensation of warmth, or it may be increased until mild warmth is felt, then reduced to the point at which the sensation is no longer perceptible. The duration of the treatment is limited to 5 to 10 minutes, and progression of the dose made cautiously according to the effects observed. When the inflammation is within a confined space, such as the air sinuses of the face, it is particularly important that excess treatment should be avoided, as rise in tension in such an area seriously aggravates the symptoms.

Dangers and Precautions

Burns. Heat burns can be caused by short-wave diathermy. In severe cases there is coagulation, and therefore destruction of the tissues, and the burn appears as a white patch surrounded by a reddened area of inflammation. In milder cases tissue is not destroyed, but a bright red patch is seen and blistering is liable to occur. The damage should be visible on removing the electrodes; it is only in exceptional circumstances that the deep tissues are raised to a higher temperature than the superficial ones, and so damage to the skin is, as a rule, apparent. Burns may arise from various causes:

(1) *Concentration of the Electric Field.* This causes overheating of the tissues in the affected area. It may be due to the presence of a small area of material of high dielectric constant within the field, such as metal or a localised patch of moisture, to inadequate electrode spacing over a prominent area of tissue, or to an electrode being badly placed so that one part of it lies nearer to the tissues than the remainder.

Metal may be embedded in the tissues, *e.g.* a plated fracture, and the danger varies with the position in which the metal lies. It is the concentration of the electric field, not overheating of the metal, that is dangerous, and if a narrow strip of metal lies parallel to the lines of force it provides a pathway of low impedance for a considerable distance, and is liable to cause serious concentration of the field (Fig. 173A). If, however, it lies across the field (Fig. 173B), the easier pathway is provided only for a short distance, and being wider than in the preceding example, it is much less likely to cause concentration of the lines of force. It is possible to calculate the degree of concentration that will occur, and the consequent danger, but the decision whether or not it is safe to apply short-wave diathermy lies with the medical officer rather than with the physiotherapist.

(2) *Excess Current.* The patient's sensation is the only indication of the intensity of the application, and excess current may be applied if he does not understand the sensations that he should experience, if cutaneous sensation is defective or if he should fall asleep during treatment. If the intensity of the

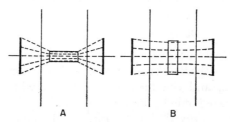

A   B

FIG. 173.—EFFECT OF METAL ON DISTRIBUTION OF ELECTRIC FIELD.

current is increased quickly at the beginning of the treatment a dangerous level may be reached, and failure to reduce the current immediately if the heat becomes intense may result in a burn occurring.

(3) *Hypersensitive Skin.* If the skin has been rendered hypersensitive, as by X-ray therapy or the recent use of liniment, a dose which would normally be safe may cause damage.

(4) *Impaired Blood Flow.* The blood circulating through the tissues normally dissipates the heat and prevents excessive rise of temperature. Should the blood flow be impaired, *e.g.* by pressure, especially on a bony point, a burn is liable to occur.

(5) *Leads Touching the Skin.* If a lead approaches close to the patient's tissues, heat is produced in the area and may be sufficient to cause a burn.

If a burn does occur, it must be reported immediately to the medical officer and also, in view of the possibility of subsequent legal proceedings, to the appropriate hospital authority. The burn must be kept clean and dry, usually being protected with a dry sterile dressing. If destruction of tissue has occurred healing will be by second intention and, as for ulcers due to other causes, various forms of physiotherapy may be used to accelerate healing, *e.g.* infra-red or ultra-violet irradiation, short-wave diathermy.

SCALDS. A scald is caused by moist heat, and may occur if the area being treated is damp, *e.g.* from perspiration, or if damp towels are used for treatment with the cable. If the moisture is not localised it does not cause concentration of the field, but may become overheated, so scalding the skin.

OVERDOSE. This causes an increase in symptoms, especially pain, and is most liable to occur when there is acute inflammation within a confined space. It can occur under other circumstances and any increase in pain following treatment is an indication to reduce the intensity of subsequent applications.

PRECIPITATION OF GANGRENE. Heat accelerates chemical changes, and therefore metabolic processes in the tissues, so increasing the demand for oxygen. Normally this is supplied by the increased blood flow, but should there be some impedance of the flow of arterial blood to the tissues the demand for oxygen is not met and gangrene is liable to develop. Consequently heat should never be applied directly to an area with an impaired arterial blood supply.

SHOCK. A shock could occur if contact were made with the apparatus circuit with the current switched on, but the construction of modern apparatus is usually such that this is not possible. Under certain circumstances a shock could result from contact with the casing of the apparatus. This is explained in Chapters 8 and 12.

SPARKING. This is liable to occur if one of the electrodes is touched while the current is applied, and the danger is considerably increased if the insulation covering the electrode is defective. Sparking may also occur on touching other metal objects in the vicinity, such as the casing of the machine, which have been charged by induction, or on touching the patient during the treatment. The reasons for sparking are explained in Chapter 12.

FAINTNESS. Faintness is produced by anæmia of the brain following a fall in blood-pressure. It is particularly liable to occur if, after an extensive treatment, the patient rises suddenly from the reclining to the erect position.

GIDDINESS. Any electrical current, when applied to the head, may cause giddiness from its effects on the contents of the semicircular canals. All diathermic treatments to the head should be given with the patient fully supported and, if possible, with the head in a horizontal or an erect position.

CHILL. During extensive treatments there is a slight rise in body temperature, and if the patient goes outside immediately after such a treatment a chill may result.

DAMAGE TO EQUIPMENT. As mentioned previously, the action of cardiac pace-makers, hearing aids and other electronic devices may be affected by disturbances set up by the short-wave diathermic current. Patients with such devices should not be treated with short-wave diathermy or allowed to come in close proximity to the apparatus. Altered action has been reported at up to six feet from the short-wave diathermic machine.

Leads may be damaged by overheating if they are allowed to make contact with a conductor, and should there be a break in the continuity of the wire, or a crack in an electrode, sparking may occur with consequent overheating. The fault may not be apparent if the insulation covering the metal is undamaged, and particular care should be taken with the malleable electrodes, which are liable to crack within their rubber covering.

Treatments should not be carried out with the patient resting on an interior sprung mattress, as sparking between the springs may be sufficient to ignite the mattress.

Contraindications

HÆMORRHAGE. The heating of the tissues by the diathermic current causes dilatation of blood-vessels, so it should not be employed directly after an injury or in any case where hæmorrhage has recently occurred. It should not be applied to the abdomen or pelvis during menstruation, nor should it be used for conditions in which hæmorrhage might occur, such as gastric or intestinal diseases associated with ulceration.

VENOUS THROMBOSIS OR PHLEBITIS. These conditions contraindicate the application of short-wave diathermy to the area drained by the affected vessel, as the increased flow of blood may dislodge the clot or aggravate the inflammation.

ARTERIAL DISEASE. As explained above, diathermy should not be applied to parts which have a defective arterial blood supply.

PREGNANCY. Diathermy should not be applied to the abdomen or pelvis during pregnancy.

METAL IN THE TISSUES may be a contraindication, depending on the position in which it lies.

LOSS OF SKIN SENSATION. It is safer to avoid the application of diathermy to areas where there is loss of skin sensation.

TUMOURS. Short-wave diathermy should not be applied in the region of malignant growths.

X-RAY THERAPY. This devitalises the tissues and renders them more susceptible to damage. So short-wave diathermy should not be applied to areas recently exposed to therapeutic doses of X-rays.

CERTAIN PATIENTS. It is unsafe to apply short-wave diathermy to patients who are unable to understand the degree of heating required and the necessity of reporting if it should become excessive. For this reason small children and mental defectives are not suitable for treatment. Similarly it is not safe to treat unconscious patients, or those who are liable to lose consciousness, such as epileptics.

PART III

ACTINOTHERAPY
AND OTHER RADIATIONS

21

PHYSICS OF HEAT AND RADIATIONS

Heat and Temperature

HEAT. Heat is a form of energy associated with vibration of molecules. Molecules are always in a state of motion, which is increased as a body gains heat and reduced as it loses heat. The motion would cease only if the body were devoid of heat energy.

TEMPERATURE. Temperature is the thermal condition of a body which determines the interchange of heat between it and other bodies. It may be regarded as the level of heat, as heat tends to pass from an object at a high temperature to an object at a lower temperature, in the same way that water tends to flow from a high level to a lower level. The temperature of a body depends on the quantity of heat that it contains and on its thermal capacity, or ability to hold the heat. When a kettle is half full of water a certain amount of heat is required to raise the temperature of the water to boiling point, but when the kettle is full of water a greater quantity of heat is required to raise the temperature to the same level, as the thermal capacity is greater. The temperature can be measured in the following scales:

(1) Centigrade .. .. 0° C. Freezing point of water at normal pressure.
100° C. Boiling point of water at normal pressure.

The interval is divided into 100 degrees.

(2) Fahrenheit .. .. 32° F. Freezing point of water at normal pressure.
212° F. Boiling point of water at normal pressure.

The interval is divided into 180 degrees.

$$F = \left(\frac{C}{5} \times 9\right) + 32$$

To calculate a temperature in Fahrenheit from Centigrade, the Centigrade temperature is divided by five and multiplied by nine, then thirty-two is added. To calculate a temperature in Centigrade from Fahrenheit, thirty-two is subtracted from the Fahrenheit temperature, then the resulting figure divided by nine and multiplied by five. $C = \dfrac{(F-32)}{9} \times 5$

(3) The Absolute Scale   273° A.   Freezing point of water at normal pressure.
373° A.   Boiling point of water at normal pressure.

In the absolute scale the degrees are the same value as in the Centigrade scale, but 0° A. is the theoretical temperature at which a body would be devoid of all heat.

MEASUREMENT OF HEAT. The unit for measuring the quantity of heat is taken as that amount of heat necessary to raise the temperature of a body of unit weight by unit amount.

One calorie is the amount of heat required to raise the temperature of 1 gramme of water through 1° C.

The British Thermal Unit (B.Th.U.) is the amount of heat required to raise the temperature of 1 lb. of water through 1° F.

THE SPECIFIC HEAT of a substance is the quantity of heat required to raise the temperature of 1 gramme of that substance through 1° C.

Physical Effects of Heat

(1) EXPANSION. When an object is heated the molecules vibrate more vigorously and fly further apart. Thus the object expands. The one exception is water, which contracts on heating between 0° C. and 4° C. The amount of expansion produced by a certain rise in temperature differs for different materials, and is indicated by the coefficient of expansion.

The Coefficient of Linear Expansion is the increase in length per unit length of a solid when the temperature is raised from 0° to 1° C.

Examples: Copper, $0 \cdot 1678 \times 10^{-4}$; invar (36 per cent. nickel, 64 per cent. steel), $0 \cdot 0087 \times 10^{-4}$; fused silica (quartz), $0 \cdot 0050 \times 10^{-4}$.

The Coefficient of Cubical Expansion is the increase in volume per unit volume when the temperature of the body is raised from 0° to 1° C.

(2) CHANGE OF STATE. Heat may cause a solid to change into a liquid, a liquid into a gas. The change of state is due to the molecules flying further apart as their vibration is increased. A considerable amount of heat is necessary to bring about the change of state, and does not cause a change of temperature.

The latent heat of a substance is the heat required to change the state of the substance without raising the temperature. For instance, the latent heat of fusion of ice is the quantity of heat required to convert unit quantity of ice into water at the same temperature. The latent heat of fusion of ice is 80 calories per gramme, that of vaporisation of water 540 calories per gramme. A corresponding amount of heat is liberated as the substance changes from a gas to a liquid or from a liquid to a solid, and the heat given off as liquid wax solidifies is utilised for treatment purposes.

(3) ACCELERATION OF CHEMICAL ACTION. Van't Hoff's law states that any chemical action capable of being accelerated by heat is accelerated by rise in temperature.

(4) PRODUCTION OF A DIFFERENCE OF POTENTIAL. If strips of two dissimilar metals are joined, and the junction is heated, a difference of potential is set up between their free ends.

(5) PRODUCTION OF ELECTROMAGNETIC WAVES. When an object is heated the increased vibration of the molecules causes displacement of electrons from one orbit to another. As the electrons return to their original orbits, energy is released, the ether is disturbed and electromagnetic waves are set up. These are infra-red, visible or ultra-violet rays and are considered more fully below (page 276).

(6) THERMIONIC EMISSION. The agitation of molecules which occurs on heating disturbs the electrons and some of them may leave the surface of the object before dropping back. They form a continually moving cloud around the object and the phenomenon is termed thermionic emission. Electrons are

emitted more readily from some materials than others, and more readily from a curved surface than from a flat one, as the former has more surface atoms than the latter. The emission occurs most easily in a vacuum, where there is no pressure to hinder the electron movement. The process is utilised in the thermionic valve, where electrons are emitted from the hot filament.

(7) REDUCED VISCOSITY OF FLUIDS. Fluids exhibit to a varying degree the property of viscosity or "stickiness", due to friction between the different layers as they move on each other. Heat reduces this effect and renders the fluid less viscid.

Transmission of Heat

Heat may be transferred from one place to another by *conduction, convection* or *radiation*.

CONDUCTION. Heat is transmitted by conduction between objects which are in contact with each other, and between different parts of one object. If two parts of an object are at different temperatures the molecules in one area are vibrating more vigorously than the molecules in the other area. The vigorously moving molecules jostle the others, causing them to vibrate more vigorously, but losing some of their own energy in doing so. Thus heat is transmitted from one part of the object to the other. The process occurs more readily in some materials than others, metals being good conductors while wood is a poor conductor of heat.

CONVECTION. Heat is transmitted by convection in a liquid or a gas. If one part of the fluid is heated, the molecules

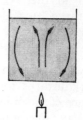

FIG. 174.—CONVECTION CURRENTS IN A FLUID.

in this area vibrate more vigorously and fly further apart. Thus the fluid expands and its density becomes less than that of the unheated fluid. The less dense fluid rises and cooler, more dense fluid takes its place. Thus convection currents are set up, and transfer the heat from one part of the fluid to another (Fig. 174).

RADIATION. A hot object emits infra-red, and possibly also visible and ultra-violet rays, which travel away from the point at which they are produced until they encounter some medium which absorbs them. When infra-red or the longer visible rays are absorbed heat is produced. Thus heat is transmitted by radiation from the object where the rays originate to the one which absorbs them. The rays produce no effects until they are absorbed, so they do not heat the intervening medium.

Radiant Energy

Radiant energy is energy in the form of waves, or rays, in the ether. The ether is an all-pervading medium which is not perceptible to any of our senses and which is presumed to exist throughout the universe. Waves are set up in the ether by movement of electrons and are known as electromagnetic waves.

WAVE-LENGTH, VELOCITY AND FREQUENCY. The wave-length of a ray is the horizontal distance from a point on one wave to the same point on the next wave (Fig. 175). The unit commonly used for measuring wave-length is the Ångström unit, which is one ten-millionth of a millimetre, and the wave-lengths of electromagnetic waves range from several kilometres to a fraction of an Ångström unit.

Electromagnetic waves travel in straight lines with a velocity of 186,326 miles, or 300,000 kilometres, per second.

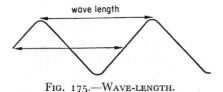

wave length

FIG. 175.—WAVE-LENGTH.

One cycle is the sequence of events that takes place between a point on one wave and the same point on the next wave, and the frequency is the number of cycles which occur in unit time. As the wave-length is the distance travelled by a wave in the course of one cycle, the product of wave-length and frequency gives the distance travelled by the wave in unit time, *i.e.* the velocity. Thus:

$$\text{Velocity} = \text{Frequency} \times \text{Wave-length}.$$

The velocity is constant for all electromagnetic waves, so the frequency varies inversely with the wave-length. The two waves shown in Fig. 176 take the same time to travel from A to

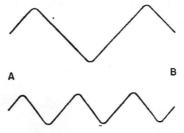

FIG. 176.—DIAGRAM TO SHOW RELATIONSHIP BETWEEN WAVE-LENGTH AND FREQUENCY.

B, but as the lower one has a shorter wave-length than the upper, it requires more cycles to cover this distance, and so has a higher frequency. When either the wave-length or the frequency is known, the other can be calculated. A high-frequency current may produce wireless waves with a wave-length of 30 metres and a frequency of 10 million cycles per second or with a wave-length of 6 metres and a frequency of 50 million cycles per second. In each case the product of frequency and wave-length is 300 million metres, or 300,000 kilometres per second.

THE ELECTROMAGNETIC SPECTRUM. The wave-lengths of electromagnetic waves vary considerably, and waves of different wave-lengths have somewhat different properties. An analysis of rays is termed a spectrum, and the electromagnetic spectrum is an analysis of the electromagnetic waves and arrangement of them according to their wavelengths and properties (Fig. 177). The rays of the electromagnetic spectrum are:

   (1) Wireless waves ..   .. Kilometres to 1,000,000 Å.
   (2) Infra-red rays   ..   .. 4,000,000 to 7,700 Å.
   (3) Visible rays   ..   .. 7,700 to 3,900 Å.
   (4) Ultra-violet rays ..   .. 3,900 to 136 Å.
   (5) X-rays ..   ..   .. 1,019 to 0·06 Å.
   (6) Gamma rays   ..   .. Up to 1·4 Å.

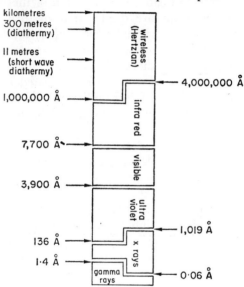

FIG. 177.—ELECTROMAGNETIC SPECTRUM.

PRODUCTION AND PROPERTIES OF ELECTROMAGNETIC WAVES. All electromagnetic waves are produced by movement of electrons, but different electron movements produce rays of different wave-lengths. The rays travel through the ether until they encounter a medium which absorbs them, and when they are absorbed the radiant energy is converted into some other form of energy and certain effects are produced. The *Law of Grotthus* states that *rays must be absorbed to produce their effects*. The effects are produced at the point at which the rays are absorbed.

Wireless, or Hertzian waves are produced by high-frequency oscillating currents and have the same frequency as the current which produces them. When the waves are absorbed by a second circuit which is in tune with the one from which they were produced, similar oscillating currents are set up (Chapter 17). Wireless waves are absorbed by metal, hence the metal screen which may be used to prevent their emission from high-frequency apparatus.

Infra-red, Visible and Ultra-violet rays are produced by heat. When a substance is heated the vibration of the molecules is increased and electrons are displaced from their orbits. As electrons return to their original orbits, energy is released. The ether is disturbed and electromagnetic waves are set up. The greater the heating, the shorter is the wavelength of the rays which are produced. When a poker is heated in the fire it becomes hot and gives off infra-red rays. If the heating is continued some visible rays are produced in addition to the infra-red rays and the poker becomes red hot. Prolonged heating renders the poker white hot, and at this stage infra-red, visible and some ultra-violet rays are emitted.

Rays of these three types are not very penetrating and are absorbed by many materials.

Infra-red rays produce heat when they are absorbed.

Visible rays, which are light rays, pass only through materials which are transparent. When visible rays are absorbed by the retina of the eye they give rise to the sensation of sight, the colour of the light depending on the wave-length of the rays. The red rays have the greatest wave-length, then orange, yellow, green, blue, indigo and violet, which have the shortest wave-length. The rays at the red end of the spectrum produce heat when they are absorbed and those at the violet end produce chemical reactions, such as the effects on photographic films.

Ultra-violet rays are absorbed to some extent by the atmosphere, also by any impurities which it may contain. When ultra-violet rays are absorbed they produce chemical reactions, such as the fading of certain dyes, effects on photographic films, and, in the skin, the conversion of 7-dehydrocholesterol into vitamin D.

X-rays are produced by passing a high voltage current through a vacuum tube, the rays being set up by the sudden stopping of the electrons at the anode.

Gamma rays are emitted as changes take place in the structure of atoms of radio-active materials.

Both these types of rays are very penetrating and when they are absorbed they produce chemical reactions. These reactions may destroy cells in the body and they produce effects on photographic films.

Laws Governing Radiations

Infra-red, visible and ultra-violet rays obey the laws of refraction, reflection, and absorption, and also the law of inverse squares.

When a beam of light encounters a different medium from the one in which it has been travelling, the rays may be absorbed by the new medium, they may be reflected by it or they may continue to travel through it. If they penetrate the new medium they may be refracted as they pass from one medium to the other.

REFRACTION. When a beam of light passes from one medium to another the rays are bent, or refracted, unless they strike the new surface at a right angle, in which case they continue to travel in the same straight line. They bend towards the normal when passing from a less dense to a denser medium, as from air to glass, and away from the normal when passing from the denser to the less dense medium, as from glass to air (Fig. 178). The normal is a line drawn perpendicular to the surface at the point where the ray strikes the new medium. The rays bend to a different extent according to their wave-length

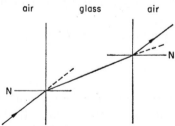

FIG. 178.—REFRACTION.

and to the relative densities of the two media. The shorter rays bend more than the longer, and the greater the difference between the densities of the media, the greater is the refraction.

If a ray is passed through a thick piece of glass with parallel surfaces, it bends in one direction on entering the glass, and back an equal amount on leaving. The emergent ray is there-

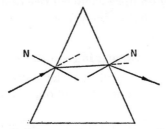

FIG. 179.—REFRACTION THROUGH A PRISM.

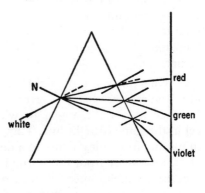

FIG. 180.—REFRACTION OF WHITE LIGHT THROUGH A PRISM.

fore parallel to the incident ray, but not in the same straight line (Fig. 178).

When a ray is passed through a prism, which is triangular in section, so that its sides are not parallel, the ray leaving the glass travels in a different direction from the one entering it (Fig. 179). If a beam of white light is passed through a prism the rays are separated, since the rays of different wave-lengths bend to a different extent (Fig. 180). If these rays fall on a screen, it is seen that the white light has been split up into the seven primary colours—red, orange, yellow, green, blue indigo and violet.

This principle is applied in the spectroscope, which is an apparatus for analysing rays. A beam of light is passed through a slit, then through a prism where it is broken up into its component parts, and finally is directed on to a screen. A spectroscope for ultra-violet rays has a quartz prism, and the screen beyond the violet end of the visible spectrum is painted with some substance such as fluorescein, which converts invisible ultra-violet rays into visible rays so that their position can be seen.

REFLECTION. When a ray strikes a new medium, it may be reflected, or turned back, from the surface. When this occurs *the angle of the incident ray to normal is equal to the angle of the reflected ray to normal* (Fig. 181).

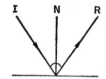

FIG. 181.—REFLECTION.

When a group of rays strikes a surface the proportion that are reflected depends on the angle at which the rays strike the surface, on the nature of the surface and on the wave-length of the rays. More rays are reflected from mirrors and bright polished surfaces than from dull or dark surfaces, and a material of a particular colour reflects only the rays of that colour. The effect of the angle at which the rays strike the surface is considered under the heading of absorption.

Reflectors may be of various shapes, and the shape of the reflector determines the behaviour of a group of rays which strikes it. When a beam of parallel rays strikes a concave reflector, the reflected rays converge. If the reflector is a gently curved section of a sphere the reflected rays all pass through a focal point in front of the reflector (Fig. 182), and if a point source of rays is placed at the focal point the rays which strike the reflector emerge parallel to each other. If, however, a beam of parallel rays strikes a deeply concave spherical reflector only those rays which strike the reflector near its centre are reflected through the focal point (Fig. 183). Thus, if a point source of rays is placed at the focal point of such a reflector, the reflected rays are not all parallel to each other. The irregular arrangement of the reflected rays may lead to undue concentration of the rays at some points, and renders the reflector unsatisfactory for treatment purposes. The reflectors used for

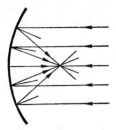

FIG. 182.—REFLECTION WITH A GENTLY CURVED
SPHERICAL REFLECTOR.

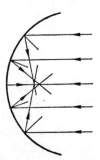

FIG. 183.—REFLECTION WITH A DEEPLY CONCAVE
SPHERICAL REFLECTOR.

infra-red and ultra-violet lamps are frequently parabolic in shape, a parabola being the shape of the section obtained on cutting through a cone parallel to its surface. The behaviour, of rays striking a parabolic reflector is shown in Fig. 184. If parallel rays strike the reflector each ray is reflected twice, all the rays pass through the focal point, and the rays finally leaving the reflector are parallel to each other. If a point source of rays is placed at the focal point, the reflected rays are parallel. These reflected rays, however, form only a small proportion of the total emitted from the generator, the majority coming directly from the source and diverging from each other. Thus radiations from a lamp with a parabolic reflector usually obey the law of inverse squares, the purpose of the parabolic reflector being to avoid the uneven distribution of rays that is liable to occur with a spherical reflector.

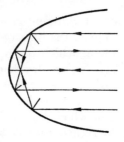

FIG. 184.—REFLECTION WITH A PARABOLIC REFLECTOR.

INTERNAL REFLECTION. If a ray strikes the surface of a new medium, which it would normally penetrate, obliquely, the angle of refraction may be such that the ray is turned back into the original medium (Fig. 185). The ray then obeys the laws of reflection and the phenomenon is known as internal reflection. It may be observed in some of the quartz rods used with the Kromayer lamp. Rays from the lamp pass down the

FIG. 185.—INTERNAL REFLECTION.

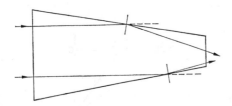

FIG. 186.—INTERNAL REFLECTION IN A QUARTZ
ROD.

rod and, if its sides slope in a certain way, are turned back into the rod whenever they tend to leave it (Fig. 186). Thus all the rays emerge from the end of the rod, none from its sides.

ABSORPTION. When rays strike the surface of a new medium some may be absorbed by the new medium, and the proportion of rays absorbed depends on the nature of the medium, the wave-length of the rays and the angle at which they strike the surface.

Different materials absorb different groups of rays, allowing others to pass through. This is the basis of filters (Chapter 23).

The effect of the angle at which the rays strike the surface is stated in the *Cosine Law*. This states that *the proportion of rays absorbed varies with the cosine of the angle between the incident ray and normal*. The cosine of an angle is determined by completing a right angled triangle, of which the angle in question forms one angle, and taking the ratio of the side adjacent to the angle to the hypotenuse. In Fig. 187:

$$\text{Cos} {<} \text{ABC} = \frac{\text{CB}}{\text{AB}}$$

$$\text{Cos} {<} \text{A}_1\text{BC} = \frac{\text{CB}}{\text{A}_1\text{B}}$$

A_1B is greater than AB

Therefore Cos ${<}$ABC is greater than Cos ${<}\text{A}_1$BC.

Thus the larger the angle, the smaller is its cosine, and if a group of rays travelling along the line AB strike the surface, a greater proportion are absorbed than would be the case if they were travelling along the line A_1B. Rays travelling along the line CB strike the surface at an angle of 90°. The angle of incidence is zero and its cosine is $\frac{\text{CB}}{\text{CB}}$, *i.e.* 1. This is the largest

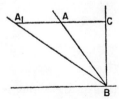

FIG. 187.—THE COSINE OF THE ANGLE OF INCIDENCE.

possible value for the cosine of an angle, and maximum absorption takes place when the rays strike the surface at a right angle.

The cosine decreases as the angle increases, but not in direct proportion to the size of the angle.

$$\text{Cos } 0° = 1. \quad \text{Cos } 60° = \tfrac{1}{2}. \quad \text{Cos } 90° = 0.$$

The number of rays that are reflected varies inversely with the number which are absorbed, so minimum reflection occurs when rays strike an object at a right angle. The greater the angle between the incident ray and normal, the greater the amount of rays which are reflected, and the smaller the amount absorbed. This law is of great importance in the application of infra-red and ultra-violet rays. The lamp and patient should be arranged so that the rays strike the skin at a right angle, thus giving maximum absorption.

In accordance with the Law of Grotthus, rays must be absorbed in order to produce an effect. When a ray is absorbed, it disappears, but produces its characteristic effects at the point where it is absorbed. Sometimes the absorption of rays is followed by the emission of rays of a longer wave-length.

FLUORESCENCE. This is an example of the above phenomenon, ultra-violet rays being absorbed and visible rays emitted. Fluorescence can be demonstrated by placing a filter which transmits only ultra-violet rays over the window of the Kromayer lamp in a dark room. A solution of quinine gives a blue fluorescence, sodium salicylate violet, and fluorescein green. Many detergents contain some fluorescent material and certain parts of the human body, such as the nails and teeth, fluoresce when exposed to ultra-violet rays. The spores of ringworm have the property of fluorescence, which is sometimes utilised in the diagnosis of this condition.

PHOSPHORESCENCE. This is shown by certain substances, including phosphorus, and is due to chemical action. Light is given off gradually and seen in the dark.

THE LAW OF INVERSE SQUARES. *The intensity of rays from a point source varies inversely with the square of the distance from the source.* Rays travelling away from a point source diverge, and at 2 feet from the source any two rays will be twice as far apart as they were at 1 foot from the source (Fig. 188). If a certain group of rays cover a square with sides 1 inch in length at 1 foot from the source, at 2 feet the same group of rays cover a square each side of which is 2 inches in length. This has four times the area of the square which they covered at 1 foot, and

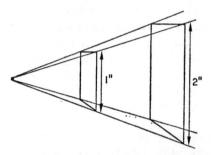

FIG. 188.—THE LAW OF INVERSE SQUARES.

so the intensity of rays at 2 feet from the source is a quarter of that at 1 foot. Similarly the intensity at 3 feet is one-ninth of the intensity at 1 foot. This law applies to infra-red, visible and ultra-violet rays, so when a lamp obeys the law of inverse squares, four minutes at 2 feet and nine minutes at 3 feet are required to produce the same effect as one minute at 1 foot. Whether a lamp obeys the law of inverse squares or not depends on the size of the source of rays, as the law is true only of rays from a point source. If a reflector is used, the divergence of the rays is reduced, but the law forms a satisfactory basis for the calculation of doses at different distances from the majority of the lamps used in a physiotherapy department.

22

INFRA-RED RAYS — *superficial heat*

INFRA-RED rays are electromagnetic waves with wave-
lengths of between 4,000,000 and 7,000 Å. They are given
off from any hot body, the greater the heating the shorter
being the wave-length of the rays emitted. The rays travel
through the ether until they encounter some medium which
absorbs them, and when they are absorbed heat is produced.

Infra-red Generators

Any hot body emits infra-red rays, so there are many sources
of these rays, such as the sun, gas, coal and electric fires, hot
water pipes, etc. Various types of generator are employed in
the physiotherapy department, but they can be divided into
two main groups, the non-luminous and the luminous generators. The former provide infra-red rays only, while the latter
emit visible and a few ultra-violet rays as well as the infra-red.
Treatment with the luminous generator is often referred to as
"radiant heat", the term "infra-red" being applied to the
radiations from the non-luminous sources. In fact these terms
are misleading as it is the infra-red rays that are utilised with
both types of generator, and both emit heat-producing rays.

NON-LUMINOUS GENERATORS. A simple type of element
for producing infra-red rays consists of a coil of wire wound on a
cylinder of some insulating material, such as fireclay or porcelain, being similar in construction to the element of an electric
radiator. An electric current is passed through the wires and
produces heat. Infra-red rays are emitted from the hot wires
and from the fireclay former, which is heated by conduction.
Some visible rays are produced as well as the infra-red and
when the element is hot a red glow is visible, so this type of
element is not perfectly non-luminous. More usually the coil of

wire is embedded in the fireclay or placed behind a plate of this material. The emission of rays is then entirely from the fireclay, which is commonly painted black, and very few visible rays are produced. Both types of element are connected into the circuit by a screw cap device and placed at the focal point of a parabolic or gently curved spherical reflector. The reflector is mounted on a stand and its position can be adjusted as required.

A third type of non-luminous generator consists of a steel tube approximately $\frac{1}{8}$ inch in diameter, within which is a spiral of wire embedded in some electrical insulator which is a good conductor of heat. Current is passed through the central wire and produces heat, which is conducted by the insulator to the steel tube, from which infra-red rays are emitted. The tube is bent into two or three large turns and mounted in a suitable reflector.

All non-luminous elements require some time to heat up and for the emission of rays to reach maximum intensity. Elements of the first type described, which emit rays directly from the wires, require about 5 minutes, but the others need longer, 10 to 15 minutes according to the construction. Lamps must therefore be switched on an appropriate time before they are required.

The construction of all lamps should be such that the reflectors and other parts do not become unduly hot during use, and it is an advantage if a wire guard prevents inadvertent contact with the element.

The non-luminous elements produce infra-red rays with wavelengths between 150,000 and 7,700 Å, or less if some visible rays are emitted. The maximum emission of rays is in the region of 40,000 Å. The small elements consume 500 watts and can be used on light circuits, but the larger ones use 750 to 1,000 watts and should be connected to power circuits.

Luminous Generators. The rays emitted from the luminous generators are produced by one or more incandescent lamps. An incandescent lamp consists of a wire filament enclosed in a glass bulb, which may be evacuated or contain an inert gas at a low pressure. The filament is a coil of fine wire and is usually made of tungsten, as this material tolerates the repeated heating and cooling. The exclusion of air prevents oxidation of the filament, which would cause an opaque deposit to form on the inside of the bulb. The wattage of bulbs used in infra-red generators may vary from 60 to 1,000, although it is now considered inadvisable to use those of higher wattage, as there is a danger that they may explode during treatment. If a bulb which consumes 300 watts or more is used, a fine mesh wire guard must be fixed across the front of the reflector. Should the bulb explode, this serves to catch a large proportion of the glass. Lamps using 150 watts or less are connected to the source of supply by a spring socket, similar to that used for electric light fittings, but larger ones have a screw cap connection. The passage of an electric current through the filament produces heat, and infra-red, visible and a few ultra-violet rays are emitted. The spectrum is from 40,000 to 3,500 Å, the greatest proportion of rays having wave-lengths in the region of 10,000 Å.

Incandescent bulbs may be mounted in various types of reflector. Tunnel baths contain a number of bulbs mounted in a semicircular metal framework. Sixty watt bulbs are commonly used and they are wired in parallel with each other, switches being provided so that some or all of the bulbs may be included in the circuit. The tunnels are made in various sizes, for treatment of different parts of the body. Alternatively a single bulb may be mounted in a parabolic reflector and bulbs of various sizes are used in this way. Incandescent bulbs may also be used in generators designed for the treatment of particular areas, such as the hand, and in the cabinet bath for irradiation of the whole body.

ACCESSORIES. Localisers can be fitted to some types of lamp and facilitate the treatment of areas of various sizes. Filters may be available and of these the most useful is the red glass filter which absorbs the shorter visible and the ultra-violet rays. The advantage of this is considered with the effects of the rays. Some lamps have a variable resistance connected in series with the bulb or element so that the output of rays can be adjusted.

Physiological Effects

When infra-red rays are absorbed by the tissues of the body, heat is produced at the point where they are absorbed. The shorter infra-red rays (7,700-12,000 Å) penetrate to the deeper parts of the dermis, or to the subcutaneous tissues, while the longer rays (more than 12,000 Å) are absorbed in the superficial epidermis (Fig. 196, page 311). Thus the rays from the non-luminous generator, the majority of which have wave-lengths in the region of 40,000 Å, are less penetrating than those from the luminous generator, most of which have wave-lengths in the region of 10,000 Å. The luminous generator provides visible and some long ultra-violet rays in addition to the infra-red. The shorter visible and the ultra-violet rays, when absorbed, produce chemical actions, which may have a slightly irritating effect. These irritating rays can be eliminated from the spectrum of the luminous generator by the use of a red glass filter. Therefore the differences in the effects of the rays from the two sources are that the rays from the luminous generator are more penetrating, but also more liable to cause irritation of the tissues, than those from the non-luminous generator. Irradiation with rays from either source results in the production of heat in the superficial tissues, and heat is conveyed to the deeper tissues by conduction and by the circulating fluids. The effects of infra-red irradiation are those of local rise in temperature, and differ from the effects of other heat treatments, *e.g.* short-wave diathermy, only in that the heat is produced at a different level. The effects of infra-red irradiation are:

INCREASED METABOLISM. This is in accordance with Van't Hoff's law, which states that any chemical change capable of being accelerated by heat is accelerated by rise in temperature. The increase in metabolism is greatest in the region where most heat is produced, *i.e.* in the superficial tissues. As a result of the increased metabolism there is an increased demand for oxygen and foodstuffs, and an increased output of waste products, including metabolites.

VASODILATATION. There is dilatation of the capillaries and arterioles in the superficial tissues. This is due to the direct effect of the heat, to the action of the metabolites and, unless the heating is very mild, to irritation of the superficial sensory nerve endings, which causes reflex vasodilatation. Thus the flow of blood to the superficial tissues is increased, an increased supply of oxygen and foodstuffs is made available, and waste products are removed. It has been assumed that there is a corresponding dilatation of the deeper vessels and increased blood flow in the deep tissues, but it seems likely that the superficial vasodilatation is accompanied by constriction of the deeper vessels, with reduction of the quantity of blood in the deep tissues. The superficial vasolidatation causes *erythema* of the skin, which, unlike that produced by ultra-violet irradiation, appears as soon as the part becomes warm and begins to fade soon after the exposure ceases. The erythema may be mottled in appearance.

PIGMENTATION. This follows repeated exposure to infra-red rays. It is mottled in appearance, and may be observed on the legs of individuals who habitually sit close to the fire. The pigmentation arises in a different way from that which follows ultra-violet irradiation, being due to the destruction of red blood cells.

EFFECTS ON SENSORY NERVES. Mild heating appears to have a sedative effect on the sensory nerve endings, while more intense heating has an irritating effect. The irritating effect is more marked in irradiation with the luminous than with the non-luminous generator, but this is probably due to the action of the shorter visible and ultra-violet rays rather than to that of the infra-red rays.

EFFECTS ON MUSCLE TISSUE. Rise in temperature assists in inducing muscle relaxation and increases the efficiency of muscle action, the fibres contract and relax more quickly and relaxation of the antagonists permits a freer action of the prime movers.

DESTRUCTION OF TISSUE. This is liable to occur if the heating is excessive.

GENERAL RISE IN TEMPERATURE. This occurs if the treatment is extensive and prolonged. The blood in the super-

L

ficial vessels is heated, then passes to other parts of the body, causing a general rise in temperature. In association with this there may be a generalised dilatation of the superficial blood vessels, due to the effect of the heated blood on the centres concerned with regulation of body temperature.

FALL IN BLOOD PRESSURE. If there is generalised vaso-dilatation the peripheral resistance is reduced, and this causes a fall in blood pressure. Heat reduces the viscosity of the blood, and this also tends to reduce the blood pressure.

INCREASED ACTIVITY OF SWEAT GLANDS. There is reflex stimulation of the sweat glands in the area exposed to the heat, resulting from the effect of the heat on the sensory nerve endings. As the heated blood circulates throughout the body it affects the centres concerned with regulation of tem-perature, and there is increased activity of the sweat glands throughout the body. When this generalised sweating occurs there is increased elimination of waste products.

Therapeutic Effects and Uses

RELIEF OF PAIN. Infra-red irradiation is frequently an effective means of relieving pain. When the heating is mild the relief of pain is probably due to the sedative effect on the superficial sensory nerve endings. Stronger heating irritates the superficial sensory nerve endings and so relieves pain by counter-irritation. Pain may be due to the accumulation in the tissues of the "P" substance, a waste product of metabolism, and an increased flow of blood through the part removes the "P" substance and so relieves the pain. In some cases the relief of pain is probably associated with the muscle relaxation mentioned below.

Pain due to acute inflammation or recent injury is relieved most effectively by mild heating. Too intense a treatment may cause an increase in the exudation of fluid into the tissues, and so increase the pain. When pain is due to lesions of a more chronic type stronger heating is required. The irradiation should cause a comfortable warmth and the treatment last for at least thirty minutes.

MUSCLE RELAXATION. Muscles relax most readily when

the tissues are warm, and the relief of pain also facilitates relaxation. So infra-red irradiation is of value in helping to achieve muscle relaxation and for the relief of muscle spasm associated with injury or inflammation.

Because of these effects of relieving pain and inducing muscle relaxation, infra-red irradiation is frequently used as a pre-liminary to other forms of physiotherapy. Following irradiation movements can frequently be carried through a greater range than before, and the relief of pain makes it possible to perform exercises more efficiently.

INCREASED BLOOD SUPPLY. This effect is most marked in the superficial tissues, and may be used in the treatment of superficial wounds and infections. A good blood supply is essential for healing to take place, and if there is infection the increased number of white blood cells and the exudation of fluid are of assistance in destroying the bacteria.

Infra-red irradiation may be used to warm cold limbs and in an attempt to increase the blood supply in poliomyelitis and other lower motor neurone lesions, although soaking the limb in warm water is often more effective.

The treatment is frequently used for arthritic joints and other inflammatory lesions, also for the after-effects of injuries. In these cases the relief of pain and muscle spasm is undoubtedly of value, but the effect of the irradiation on the flow of blood through the site of the lesion is uncertain. When superficial structures are affected there may be some heating of, and consequent vasodilatation in, these structures, e.g. small joints of the hands and feet. This will increase the supply of oxygen and foodstuffs available to the tissues, accelerate the removal of waste products and help to bring about the resolution of inflammation. On the other hand irradiation of the skin over deeply placed structures is more likely to cause vaso-constriction in the deep tissues. This may be of value in relieving congestion.

ELIMINATION OF WASTE PRODUCTS. Extensive treat-ments cause increased activity of the sweat glands throughout the body, with increased elimination of waste products. This is of value in some cases of generalised arthritis.

Technique of Irradiation

CHOICE OF APPARATUS. In many cases the luminous and non-luminous generators are equally suitable, but in some instances one proves more satisfactory than the other. When there is acute inflammation or recent injury, the sedative effect of the rays obtained from the non-luminous generator may prove more effective for relieving pain than the counter-irritant effect of those from the luminous source. For lesions of a more chronic type the counter-irritant effect of the shorter rays may prove to be of most value, and under these circumstances a luminous generator is chosen.

The most suitable generator for the area to be treated is selected. If only one surface of the body requires irradiation a lamp with a single element mounted in a reflector is satisfactory, but if several aspects require treatment a tunnel bath is more effective. The temperature reached in the tunnel baths is higher than that produced by the other lamps and this may be an advantage, particularly for the treatment of chronic lesions.

Before use the lamp is checked to ensure that it is working correctly and a localiser or filter fitted if required. Non-luminous generators are switched on an adequate time before use.

PREPARATION OF THE PATIENT. Clothing is removed from the affected part and at the first attendance skin sensation to heat and cold is tested. Should the sensation be defective it is unwise to apply the treatment, for apart from the patient's inability to appreciate possible overheating, the vasomotor response in the affected area is likely to be less than in a normal one, so that heat is not carried away so rapidly. The patient is warned that he should experience comfortable warmth, that he should report immediately if the heating becomes excessive, and that undue heat may cause a burn; also that he should not touch the lamp or move nearer to it. The patient should be comfortable and fully supported so that he does not move unduly during treatment.

ARRANGEMENT OF THE LAMP AND PATIENT. The

lamp is arranged in position so that it is opposite to the centre of the area and the rays strike the skin at a right angle, thus ensuring maximum absorption. The distance of the lamp from the patient is measured and is usually 2 feet or 18 inches, according to the output of the generator.

Tunnel baths are placed over the part and in theory should be left open at both ends. This permits the circulation of air, so aiding the evaporation of sweat which, should it accumulate on the skin, absorbs the rays. It may, however, be found more satisfactory to cover the bath with a blanket. The air inside the tunnel then becomes warm and the patient is heated partly by radiation and partly by conduction from the hot air. A higher temperature is reached than when the ends are open and this may prove beneficial.

Care must be taken that the patient's face is not exposed to the rays and protection can be provided by a localiser or a paper shade. If it is not possible to avoid irradiating the face the eyes may be shielded with pads of damp cotton wool, as water absorbs the rays.

APPLICATION OF TREATMENT. At the commencement of the exposure the intensity of irradiation should be mild, but after 5 to 10 minutes, when vasodilatation has taken place and the increased blood flow become established, the strength of the application may be increased. This can be achieved by moving the lamp nearer to the patient, by adjusting the variable resistance or by increasing the number of bulbs used in a tunnel bath.

The physiotherapist should be at hand throughout the treatment session and reduce the intensity of the application if the heat becomes excessive. If the irradiation is extensive it is desirable that sweating should occur to counteract undue rise in body temperature, and this is encouraged if the patient is provided with water to drink during the treatment.

At the end of the exposure the skin should be red, but not excessively so. Following extensive irradiation the patient should not rise suddenly from the recumbent position, or go out into the cold immediately.

DURATION AND FREQUENCY OF TREATMENT. For

acute inflammation or recent injury and for the treatment of wounds and infections an exposure of 10 to 15 minutes is adequate, but may be applied several times during the day. Longer exposures are desirable for chronic conditions, 30 minutes being the usual duration, and the treatment can be applied once daily or on alternate days.

Dangers of Infra-red Irradiation

BURNS. Infra-red irradiation can cause superficial heat burns. A red patch is seen on the skin, which subsequently blisters, either during or after the treatment. The burn is most often caused by too great an intensity of irradiation and this can occur if the patient does not understand the nature of the treatment, fails to report overheating, moves nearer to the lamp or falls asleep during the treatment. Also if the skin sensation is defective so that the patient is unable to appreciate the degree of heating, or if the physiotherapist is not at hand to reduce the heat if necessary. Failure to allow adequate time for a non-luminous generator to warm up before placing it in position may result in overheating when the temperature of the element rises.

The recent use of liniment renders the skin hypersensitive and so increases the danger of burns. Impaired blood flow through the part, which may be due to pressure or to some circulatory defect, increases the risk of overheating, as the heat is not carried away from the area as rapidly as usual.

Burns can also occur as a result of touching the lamp when it is hot, or from the hot glass which is scattered if an incandescent bulb breaks. It is possible for blankets or pillows to catch fire, especially pillows placed carelessly in a tunnel bath.

Should a burn occur the procedure is the same as for a short-wave diathermy burn (page 261).

ELECTRIC SHOCK. This could occur as a result of touching some exposed part of the circuit, but the chief danger is that of the live wire coming in contact with the apparatus casing. This is considered in Chapter 12, and in view of the extensive metal framework of many infra-red generators it is essential that appropriate precautions are taken.

PRECIPITATION OF GANGRENE. The danger of applying infra-red rays to an area with defective arterial blood supply is the same as for short-wave diathermy.

HEADACHE. Headache may follow infra-red irradiation, especially if sweating does not occur or if the treatment is given during hot weather. The patient should take plenty of fluid to encourage sweating and it is wise to discontinue extensive infra-red treatments when the weather is very hot. Irradiation of the back of the head may cause headache and the area should be protected with a localiser or shade.

CONSTIPATION. This may result if the water lost by sweating is not replaced by increased fluid intake.

FAINTNESS. Extensive irradiation is accompanied by a fall in blood pressure which may result in faintness due to anaemia of the brain. This is particularly liable to occur if the patient rises suddenly from the recumbent position after an extensive treatment.

CHILL. Extensive irradiation is accompanied by a rise in body temperature which may be as great as $2°$ F. ($1°$ C.), and should the patient go out immediately after such a treatment a chill may result.

INJURY TO THE EYES. It has been suggested that exposure to infra-red rays may predispose to cataract, and it is wise to protect the eyes from irradiation.

Contraindications

Infra-red irradiation should not be applied to areas with a defective arterial blood supply, nor where there is danger of hæmorrhage.

It is unwise to apply the treatment to areas where the skin sensation is defective or on which liniment has recently been used.

23

THE PRODUCTION OF ULTRA-VIOLET RAYS

Transmission of Current through Gases

A GAS at atmospheric pressure is a poor conductor of electricity, but as the pressure is reduced the conductivity increases.

IONISATION OF GASES. In order that a gas may conduct an electric current it must be ionised. That is, some electrons must be displaced from their atoms, which become positive ions, the free electrons being classed as negative ions. The gas

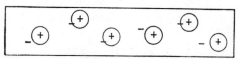

FIG. 189.—IONISED GAS.

then contains positive and negative ions in addition to neutral molecules (Fig. 189). Ionisation is brought about by various electrical disturbances, such as cosmic and other radiations, radio-activity and the electric field set up by a high voltage charge. Most gases contain a few ions, but it may be necessary to apply some additional force before the ionisation is sufficient for a current to pass.

PASSAGE OF CURRENT. When a P.D. is applied across an ionised gas, the free electrons move towards the positive electrode and the positive ions towards the negative electrode. These moving particles collide with other atoms, displacing electrons from them and increasing the ionisation of the gas. The electrons pass to the anode and on round the circuit, while the positive ions travel to the cathode where they receive electrons and are neutralised (Fig. 190). Although charged particles are lost in this way, the ionisation of the gas is maintained as the moving ions collide with neutral atoms and displace electrons from them. Thus the current continues to flow, and as it consists of a two-way movement of ions it is classed as a *convection current.* If the gas is at atmospheric pressure the molecules are crowded together and it is difficult for the particles to move, so the resistance is high. Several thousand volts are

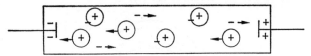

FIG. 190.—PASSAGE OF CURRENT
THROUGH A GAS.

required to pass a current across a narrow air gap at atmospheric pressure. As the pressure of the gas is reduced the molecules are less crowded and the particles can move more easily, so the resistance is reduced. If the pressure falls below a certain level the resistance rises again, as there are insufficient ions to transmit the current.

VISIBLE EFFECTS. When the charged particles recombine to form neutral molecules energy is released in the form of heat and light. A momentary passage of current causes a *spark,* and an intermittent current gives rise to a series of sparks. It is usually when the pressure of the gas is high that sparks are observed, as reduction of the pressure, and so of the resistance, results in a continuous passage of current. This sets up a luminous *glow discharge,* the colour of which is characteristic of the particular gas, being violet for air, red for neon and greenish-blue for argon. This is the principle underlying the action of tubes containing neon gas which are used as tuning indicators for short-wave diathermy. The gas within the tube is at a low pressure, and when the tube is placed in the electric field high-frequency currents are set up in the gas and cause a red glow. This reaches maximum intensity when the circuits are in tune and the field at its strongest.

If the gas through which the current passes is the vapour of some metal or carbon, a flame is formed which is termed an *electric arc*.

The Electric Arc

An electric arc is the flame produced by the passage of a current through the vapour of some metal or carbon. It is so called because, if the electrodes between which the current passes are placed horizontally, the flame curves upward in the shape of an arc of a circle (Fig. 191).

FIG. 191.—THE ELECTRIC ARC.

PRODUCTION OF AN ELECTRIC ARC. The carbon arc provides a simple example of the way in which an electric arc is produced. It is used for a variety of purposes, and in the past was extensively employed for the production of ultra-violet rays in physiotherapy departments. Nowadays it is used for treatment purposes only in some of the small home sunlight lamps. Two carbon rods are brought in contact with each other and a current passed through them. The point of contact of the rods is of small cross-sectional area, so offers a high resistance, and intense heat is generated which vapourises the carbon. The rods are then separated, the vapour fills the gap and is ionised by the P.D. between the electrodes and by the emission of electrons from the hot negative carbon (thermionic emission). Current passes through the vapour in the manner described above and the electric arc is formed, the process being known as "striking" the arc. The carbon of the electrodes is vaporised, so the rods become shorter as the arc burns.

The presence of the vapour, even at atmospheric pressure, causes a marked reduction in the resistance of the gap. Current can pass across a gap 2 or 3 inches wide on the application of a P.D. of 80 to 100 volts.

The same principles apply to the production of other types of arc. The vapour of a metal is present, this is ionised by some means and the application of a P.D. produces a current through it. An arc is liable to form whenever two metal contacts through which a current is passing are separated. For this reason switches in electrical circuits must have strong springs, which ensure sudden separation of the contacts so that an arc is not established between them.

EMISSION OF RAYS. When an electric arc is formed intense heat and illumination result, infra-red, visible and ultra-violet rays being emitted. When a metal is heated to incandescence, the spectrum of rays produced is continuous and is the same for all metals. When the metal is heated until vapour is formed it yields a spectrum which is specific for that metal and is in the form of lines or bands. For instance, if common salt is heated in a flame and the flame examined with a spectroscope in a dark room, the characteristic yellow line of sodium is seen. As the rays emitted by an electric arc are from a vapour source, the spectrum is typical of the material used and is in the form of lines. These may be superimposed on a continuous spectrum if rays are also emitted from the incandescent electrodes.

The spectrum obtained from the mercury arc is characteristic of mercury, being deficient in red and orange rays, and is in the form of lines, as it is entirely from a vapour source. That of the carbon arc is continuous with bright bands super-

	Infra-red.	Visible.	Ultra-violet.
Sunlight	20,000 to 7,700 Å. 80 per cent.	7,700 to 3,900 Å. 13 per cent.	3,900 to 2,900 Å. 7 per cent.
Plain carbon arc	20,000 to 7,700 Å. 85 per cent.	7,700 to 3,900 Å. 10 per cent.	3,900 to 2,900 Å. 5 per cent.
Mercury vapour arc	20,000 to 7,700 Å. 52 per cent.	6,000 to 3,900 Å. 20 per cent.	3,900 to 1,890 Å. 28 per cent.
Kromayer lamp	Absorbed by the water	6,000 to 3,900 Å.	3,900 to 1,849 Å.
Fluorescent tubes	20,000 to 7,700 Å.	6,000 to 3,900 Å.	3,900 to 2,800 Å.
Incandescent lamp	40,000 to 7,700 Å.	7,700 to 3,900 Å.	3,900 to 3,500 Å.
Pure infra-red lamp	150,000 to 7,700 Å.	None	None

imposed, since some of the rays are given off from the incandescent ends of the electrodes. The spectra obtained from various arc lamps are given on page 299, together with those of the sun and infra-red generators, for comparison.

Ultra-violet Lamps

Ultra-violet rays for the treatment of patients are obtained from arc lamps.

MERCURY VAPOUR LAMPS. These are used extensively for the production of ultra-violet rays for therapeutic purposes and various types of lamp are available. Electronic discharge tube burners are used in modern lamps and may be of the high- or low-pressure type. The lamp may be air- or water-cooled, and the former designed either for the treatment of individual patients or for a group.

FLUORESCENT TUBES. This type of generator is of comparatively recent development. It is designed for general irradiation, and for this purpose has certain advantages over the mercury vapour lamps. These advantages are considered with the effects of the rays.

The Air-cooled Electronic Discharge Mercury Vapour Lamp

THE BURNER. This consists of an arc tube of fused quartz, which is exhausted of air and contains a little argon gas and a few drops of mercury. An electrode is introduced into each end of the arc tube and current is led to these electrodes by metal conductors sealed into the tube, special construction being adopted to obviate loss of vacuum when the tube expands.

The tube is made of quartz because this material transmits ultra-violet rays, has a high melting point and a low co-efficient of expansion. The conductors passing through the quartz are of a material with about the same coefficient of expansion as quartz, as otherwise the seal might be broken and air enter the burner when it became hot during use. All air must be excluded from the arc tube, otherwise the heat would cause a reaction between the oxygen and the mercury resulting in the formation of oxide of mercury, which would appear as a yellowish-brown deposit on the inside of the quartz tube and interfere with the transmission of rays. The presence of some gas within the arc tube is necessary to assist in striking the arc, and argon is used because it is an inert gas which does not react with the mercury or the electrodes.

The low-pressure burner has a straight arc tube, about 5 inches in length, while that of the high-pressure burner is shorter and U-shaped. The gases in the latter are at a higher pressure, though still considerably below atmospheric pressure, and both give about the same output of rays.

THE CIRCUIT (Fig. 192). The burner is wired in series with a switch and the stabilising resistance, part of which is in

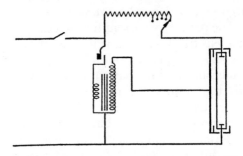

FIG. 192.—CIRCUIT OF ELECTRONIC DISCHARGE
MERCURY VAPOUR LAMP.

the form of a series rheostat and can be cut out of the circuit. In parallel with the main circuit is the starter circuit which is completed by depressing a press-button switch. This circuit contains the primary coil of a step-up autotransformer, and one end of the secondary coil of this transformer is connected to metal caps placed over the ends of the burner. The caps of the low-pressure burner are connected together by a metal strip lying beside the arc tube.

WORKING. When the switch is turned on a potential difference is set up between the electrodes, but current cannot pass across the burner until the argon is sufficiently ionised. The P.D. between the electrodes, together with electrical disturbances from outside sources, may be sufficient to ionise the argon, but more frequently the starter circuit must be employed. When the button is depressed current passes through the primary coil of the autotransformer and induces an EMF of about 600 volts in the secondary coil. This charges the metal caps over the ends of the burner and the resulting electric field displaces electrons from the atoms of the argon, so increasing the ionisation of the gas. When the argon is sufficiently ionised current passes in the manner previously described and a greenish-blue glow discharge is seen. Once the current is passing the ionisation is maintained by collisions between the particles, so the starter circuit is required only to initiate the process. The passage of the current through the argon produces heat which vapourises the mercury, the mercury vapour mixes with the argon and is ionised as moving particles collide with the atoms. The passage of current through the mercury vapour produces an electric arc, and when this is formed intense illumination results. Three to four minutes are required for the arc to be established and the output of rays to reach maximum intensity, so the lamp is turned on 5 minutes before it is required. The quantity of mercury included in the tube is such that it is all vaporised when the burner is fully operating, and as the arc is formed within a closed tube none of the vapour is lost. Consequently the amount of mercury vapour, and so the production of rays, is constant.

THE STABILISING RESISTANCE. This is included in the circuit in order to obtain the correct potential drop across the arc, the total voltage being divided between the stabilising resistance and the burner in direct proportion to their resistance. Quartz is used for the arc tube because it transmits ultra-violet rays, but heat causes the quartz gradually to change into tridymite, another form of silica. Tridymite is opaque to ultra-violet rays and as it is formed the output of rays tends to fall. To counteract this, part of the stabilising resistance is cut out of the circuit, so increasing the P.D. across the burner and the intensity of current in the circuit. The production of rays is increased, so although the proportion that passes through the arc tube is diminished the output is maintained at a constant level.

CONSTRUCTION OF THE LAMP. The lamp for the treatment of individual patients incorporates either the high- or the low-pressure burner, which is mounted at the focal point of a parabolic reflector. The reflector is supported on a stand in such a way that its position can be adjusted, and the resistances and transformer are housed in the base of the lamp.

The "Centrosol" lamp, which is designed for the treatment of a group of patients, has two low-pressure burners mounted vertically with no reflector. Thus a number of patients can sit round the lamp and receive treatment together.

CURRENT CONSUMPTION, SPECTRUM AND DOSE. When all the stabilising resistance is in the circuit the P.D. across the arc is 125 volts. When the lamp is running the intensity of current is between 2 and 4 amperes, depending on the type of lamp and the position of the rheostat control. When the starter circuit is included the current rises to 5 amperes, so the lamp must be connected to a power circuit.

The lamp provides infra-red rays with wave-lengths between 20,000 and 7,700 Å, which form 52 per cent. of the total output, visible rays with wave-lengths between 6,000 and 3,900 Å, forming 20 per cent. of the total, and ultra-violet rays with wave-lengths between 3,900 and 1,890 Å, forming the remaining 28 per cent. The spectrum is in the form of lines and is typical of mercury, there being no red or orange rays but a large proportion of the short ultra-violet rays.

The dose required varies with different lamps, but the average is 2 minutes at 3 feet for a first-degree erythema.

The Kromayer Lamp

The Kromayer lamp is a water-cooled mercury vapour lamp. It is suitable only for local irradiation, but has the advantages that it can be used in contact with the tissues or, with a suitable applicator, to irradiate the interior of the nose, mouth, throat or other cavity.

CONSTRUCTION (Fig. 193). The burner is a small U-shaped high-pressure electronic discharge tube, placed with the convexity forwards within a metal jacket which has a quartz window in front. A second metal jacket, also with a quartz window, surrounds the inner one and water circulates between the two. The outer window can be unscrewed for cleaning, or the whole front of the lamp detached (at D in Fig. 193) for freer access. The inner window can be removed if the burner requires attention or replacement.

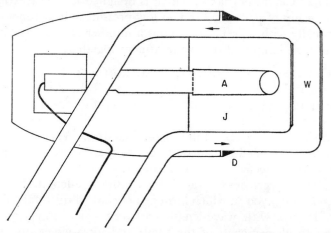

FIG. 193.—SECTION THROUGH THE KROMAYER LAMP.
W, water; A, arc tube; J, space between inner metal case and the burner.

WATER SUPPLY. The supply of cold water may come from a tap or, more commonly, distilled water may be used. The latter is stored in a tank and the water is pumped through the lamp by an electric motor. The water enters the lamp below and leaves at the top, thus keeping the space in front of the arc tube full of water. Tap water has the disadvantage that it contains salts and other impurities, which may be deposited on the quartz windows and interfere with the transmission of rays. This does not occur when distilled water is used, and the self-contained lamp has the additional advantage that it can be moved where required. The water does, however, tend to become warm with prolonged use, as the tank contains only $1\frac{1}{2}$ pints.

CIRCUIT AND WORKING. The principles of these are similar to those of the air-cooled lamp, except that a different starter circuit is used. This does not, however, affect the operation of the lamp.

The water must be circulating freely and any air bubbles eliminated, by tilting the lamp, before the burner is switched on. Five minutes are then required for the output of rays to reach full intensity. The casing of the lamp should not become unduly hot during use, and the water should be allowed to circulate for 5 minutes after the burner has been turned off, to ensure thorough cooling.

As with the air-cooled lamp, a rheostat control enables the output of rays to be maintained as the quartz changes into tridymite.

SPECTRUM AND DOSE. The spectrum is similar to that of the air-cooled lamp, except that the infra-red rays are absorbed by the water. Thus visible rays, with wave-lengths between 6,000 and 3,900 Å, form 40 per cent. of the total, the remaining 60 per cent. being ultra-violet rays with wave-lengths between 3,900 and 1,849 Å. There is a large proportion of short ultra-violet rays.

The average dose for a first-degree erythema is 2 seconds in contact or 10 seconds at 4 inches from the window of the lamp.

ACCESSORIES. Various accessories are available for use with the Kromayer lamp.

A mica cap can be fitted over the quartz window to prevent the emission of rays when the burner is operating but the lamp not in use.

A convex quartz applicator is used for compressing the tissues during treatment. The purpose of this is considered with the methods of application.

Quartz rods, which are made in various shapes and sizes, are used for the irradiation of cavities. Rays are given off only from the end of the rod. If the shape of the rod is such that there is total internal reflection, no special measures are necessary to ensure this, but if it is not of such a shape the rod is surrounded by a metal sheath which prevents the emission of rays from the sides. Some rays are absorbed by the quartz, and so a longer dose is required with the rod than when the lamp is used in contact with the tissues. The exact increase necessary differs for different rods, so each one must be tested and the necessary exposure noted as a multiple of the contact dose required to produce the same effect. An approximate assessment of the exposure can be made by adding one contact dose for each inch of rod; *e.g.* a rod 3 inches long might require 4 times the contact dose.

The convex applicator and rods are attached to the front of the lamp by a holder, which usually has a shutter to facilitate timing of the exposure.

Various filters can be used with the lamp and are included in the list at the end of the chapter.

Care of Mercury Vapour Lamps

Lamps must be kept clean, dry and free from dust.

The lamp should not be turned on and off more frequently than is necessary and should be left burning when required for further use within half an hour.

In order to maintain a constant output of rays the stabilising resistance must be adjusted when necessary. The point to which the control should be moved after a certain number of hours of burning is marked, and in order that adjustment can be made at the correct intervals a record should be kept of the time for which the lamp is in operation. After 1,000 hours of use the increased production of rays can no longer compensate for the reduced transmission by the arc tube and the burner must be renewed. It is necessary to test the output of the lamp at regular intervals, for instance, whenever the control is adjusted.

The burner of an air-cooled lamp should be cleaned regularly with absolute alcohol. Other forms of spirit contain impurities which, when the lamp is hot, become permanently etched into the quartz. The burner should not be touched with the fingers, but if this does occur the arc tube must be cleaned immediately, as grease from the fingers acts in the same way as other impurities.

The water supply of the Kromayer lamp must be operated in the manner described, as considerable damage may result from overheating. At regular intervals, *e.g.* after every eight hours of use, the distilled water should be renewed and the surfaces of the quartz windows with which it comes in contact cleaned. A clean chamois leather and the moisture remaining on the quartz should prove adequate for this, but if ineffective a special quartz cleaning material must be used, as other cleaning agents are liable to react with the material of the water pipes, and a deposit on the windows results.

Fluorescent Tubes for Ultra-violet Radiation

The mercury vapour lamp can be used for general ultra-violet irradiation but has the disadvantage that the spectrum contains a large proportion of the short ultra-violet rays, which are undesirable for general treatments. In recent years an attempt has been made to produce a lamp which provides a more suitable spectrum for this purpose.

The fluorescent tubes are similar to the tubes used for lighting. Each tube is 4 feet in length, and is made of a special type of glass which transmits more ultra-violet rays than ordinary window glass. The inner surface of the tube is coated with a special phosphor, and a low pressure mercury arc is set up within the tube. The rays produced by the arc are absorbed by the phosphor, from which rays of longer wave-lengths are emitted. The tubes emit a few infra-red rays, some of the shorter visible rays and a large proportion of the long ultra-violet rays. The rays with wave-lengths of less than 2,800 Å are absorbed by the glass. Some tubes also emit a narrow band of rays with wave-lengths in the region of 2,500 Å, but this band is absent from the spectrum of the more recent models.

THE LAMP. The tubes are intended for general irradiation, and may be arranged either for the treatment of individual patients or for a group. When designed for the latter, six tubes are placed vertically on a circular base, with no reflector, and the patients are arranged round them. A plan of this arrangement is shown in Fig. 194, the small circles in the centre representing the tubes, the larger circles, marked "P," the patients.

The lamp for treatment of individual patients has four tubes, each with a parabolic reflector, arranged in a semicircular metal frame. Two infra-red elements are included in order to keep the patient warm during treatment. The tubes are arranged so that when the lamp is a suitable distance above the patient half the body surface is irradiated. When the lamp is in the correct position all the tubes should be at 18 inches from the patient (Fig. 195). The area of skin immediately

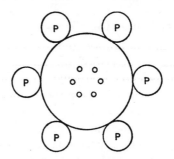

FIG. 194.—PLAN OF GROUP TREATMENT WITH FLUORESCENT TUBES.

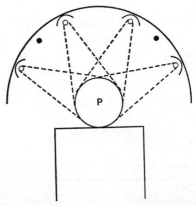

FIG. 195.—TUNNEL MODEL OF FLUORESCENT TUBES.

opposite to each tube is irradiated by rays from this tube striking the skin at right angles, and by rays from adjacent tubes striking the surface obliquely. The intermediate areas each receive rays from two tubes striking the skin somewhat obliquely. The final reaction should be relatively even over the whole surface, although irregularities may occur owing to the different shape and size of individual patients. The above explanation assumes that the patient is a cylinder 1 foot in diameter, which is rarely exactly accurate. If the patient is treated in both the prone and supine positions practically the whole surface of the body, including the sides of the trunk, is irradiated. Care must be taken that the lamp is not placed too low, or the sides of the body receive a double exposure.

DOSE. With the lamp for the treatment of individual patients, arranged as described above, the average dose is 3 minutes for a first-degree erythema. The full output of rays is obtained as soon as the lamp is turned on, and the output falls only slowly as the tubes become older.

Filters

A light filter is a substance which absorbs some rays and allows others to pass through.

(1) Window glass absorbs ultra-violet rays below 3,300 Å.

(2) Vitaglass absorbs ultra-violet rays below 2,750 Å.

(3) Water absorbs infra-red rays.

(4) Chance's Crookes A glass absorbs ultra-violet rays and is used for goggles.

(5) Blue uviol glass absorbs the abiotic rays below 2,900 Å. It also absorbs the red end of the visible spectrum. It is used to prevent irritation of the new epithelium in healing wounds. Four times the usual exposure is required.

(6) Oxide of nickel glass, Wood's filter, and Chance's ultra-violet glass are glasses which transmit ultra-violet rays only. They are used with the Kromayer or air-cooled mercury vapour lamp in a dark room to show fluorescence.

(7) Mica is used for the protective cap of the Kromayer lamp. It absorbs all the ultra-violet and some of the visible rays.

(8) Cellophane, liquid paraffin or cod-liver oil are sometimes used instead of the blue uviol filter. These substances absorb the short ultra-violet rays.

24

EFFECTS OF ULTRA-VIOLET RAYS

ULTRA-VIOLET rays are electromagnetic waves with wave-lengths of between 3,900 and 136 Å, those with wave-lengths between 3,900 and 1,849 Å being available for treatment purposes. When ultra-violet rays are absorbed chemical effects are produced.

The Skin

Ultra-violet rays are absorbed in the skin and it is there that the reactions occur which cause the beneficial effects.

The skin consists of two main layers, the epidermis and dermis, and the epidermis can be subdivided into superficial and deep layers. The deep epidermis consists of two layers. The stratum germinativum is a row of nucleated columnar cells resting on the papillæ of the dermis, and it is in this layer that the reproduction of cells takes place to replace those lost from the surface. Above this is the stratum mucosum, a mass of irregular-shaped nucleated cells (prickle cells), between which are tiny lymph channels for the nourishment of the cells. Pigment is formed in the deep epidermis.

The superficial epidermis consists of three layers, in which the nucleated cells are transformed into flat, horny cells without nuclei. The deepest layer, stratum granulosum, consists of nucleated cells which contain granules. In the stratum lucidum and the most superficial layer, the stratum corneum, the cells are flattened and have lost their nuclei. A blister following ultra-violet irradiation is caused by effusion of fluid between the stratum lucidum and the stratum granulosum and heals without a scar, since the growing layer of cells of the deep epidermis is intact, but an ulcer, where these cells are destroyed, heals by scar formation.

The dermis consists mainly of fibrous tissue and projects upwards in the form of papillæ, which contain capillary loops from the blood-vessels of the dermis. In the deeper part of the dermis are the sweat glands, whose ducts pass in a spiral manner

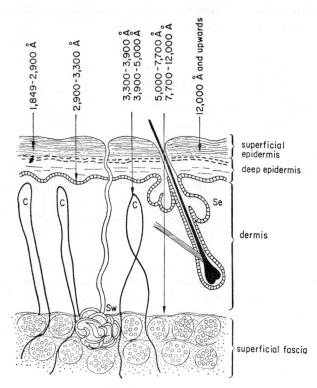

FIG. 196.—PENETRATION OF RAYS INTO SKIN.
C, capillary; Se, sebaceous gland; Sw, sweat gland.

to the surface. Hair follicles extend from the dermis to the surface of the skin, and the ducts of the sebaceous glands open into the hair follicles in the dermis. Whenever the hair is erected by contraction of the arrector pili muscle, sebum is squeezed out of the gland into the hair follicle, and so to the surface. The sebum is a fatty material which is absorbed into the superficial part of the skin and keeps it supple. Cholesterol and the associated substance 7-dehydrocholesterol are found in sebum. Nerve fibres ending in touch corpuscles and other sensory end organs are also found in the dermis. Below the dermis is the superficial fascia containing fat. The skin is between ½ and 2 millimetres in thickness, being thickest in the palms of the hands and soles of the feet.

Penetration of Rays into the Skin
(Fig. 196)

Ultra-violet rays with wave-lengths between 2,900 and 1,849 Å are absorbed in the superficial epidermis.

Ultra-violet rays with wave-lengths between 3,300 and 2,900 Å are absorbed in the deep epidermis.

Ultra-violet rays with wave-lengths between 3,900 and 3,300 Å are absorbed in the blood of the superficial capillary loops in the dermis. When compression treatment is given with the Kromayer lamp the blood is driven out of these capillaries, and in consequence the long ultra-violet rays can penetrate more deeply.

Visible rays with wave-lengths between 5,000 and 3,900 Å— the violet end of the visible spectrum—are also absorbed in the blood of the superficial capillaries of the dermis.

Visible rays with wave-lengths between 7,700 and 5,000 Å— the red end of the visible spectrum—penetrate more deeply and can actually pass through the skin. That red rays are more penetrating than other visible rays is demonstrated on foggy days, when the sun appears red.

Short infra-red rays with wave-lengths between 12,000 and 7,700 Å penetrate to the subcutaneous tissues.

Long infra-red rays with wave-lengths of more than 12,000 Å are absorbed in the superficial epidermis.

Figs. 197 and 198 show the rays which are provided by various sources, the levels at which they are absorbed and the rays which produce particular effects.

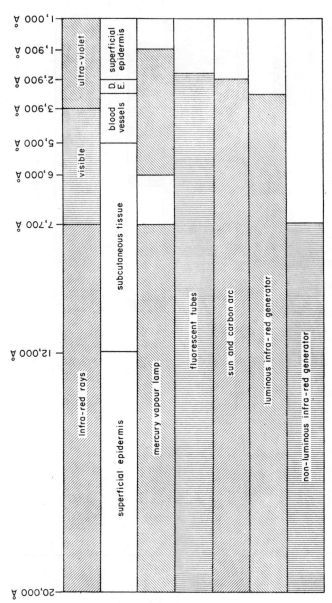

FIG. 197—SPECTRA OF LAMPS AND DEPTH OF PENETRATION OF RAYS INTO THE SKIN.

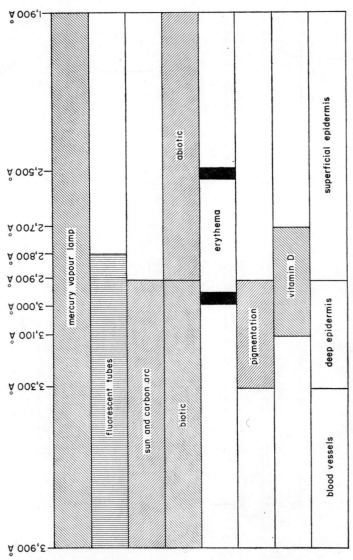

Fig. 198.—Ultra-Violet Rays Produced by Different Lamps, and Rays which produce particular effects.

Physiological Effects of Ultra-violet Rays

The effects of ultra-violet rays on the body may be divided into two groups; those which are produced locally in the area exposed to the rays, and the general effects resulting from a more widespread irradiation. The following *local effects* are produced:

ERYTHEMA REACTION. Ultra-violet rays, when absorbed in the skin, cause chemical actions which result in irritation and destruction of cells. This causes liberation of the "H" substance which produces the triple response in a similar manner to histamine. The triple response is dilatation of the capillaries, due directly to the chemical effect of the "H" substance, dilatation of arterioles, due to the axon reflex, and exudation of fluid into the tissues, due to the increased permeability of the capillary walls. These effects are similar to the changes observed in inflammation, and the erythema may be regarded as an inflammatory reaction. The intensity of the reaction varies considerably, according to the strength of the irradiation. A mild dose causes slight reddening of the skin, which is accompanied by no other symptoms and soon fades, but following a longer exposure the skin is very red, hot and sore and there is marked vasodilatation with exudation of fluid and white blood corpuscles into the skin. Œdema of the skin results, and if the exuded fluid separates the stratum lucidum from the stratum granulosum a blister is formed.

There are two groups of rays which produce the erythema reaction, one with wave-lengths in the region of 2,500 Å, the other in the region of 2,970 Å. The mode of action of these two groups of rays appears to be slightly different. Those with the shorter wave-lengths are absorbed in the superficial epidermis and cause changes in this region, which are followed by the erythema reaction. If the superficial epidermis is absent the effects of these rays are considerably reduced, so the reaction that they produce must be peculiar to the superficial epidermis, not one that can take place at any level in the tissues. Rays of the group with the longer wave-lengths are absorbed in the deep epidermis and cause a chemical reaction at this level, which again results in the production of erythema.

The effects of these rays are increased if the superficial epidermis is absent, as the rays are then able to penetrate more easily to the deeper layers.

Following exposure to ultra-violet rays, there is no immediate effect to be seen on the skin, the erythema appearing up to twelve hours after irradiation. The reaction generally becomes visible sooner after a strong dose than after a weak one. This delay in the appearance is one of the ways in which the erythema differs from that produced by infra-red rays, which appears during irradiation. Heat affects the blood-vessels directly, while the effect of ultra-violet irradiation is indirect, being the result of chemical actions initiated by the rays.

Four *degrees of erythema* are described:

(1) A first-degree erythema is a slight reddening of the skin, with no irritation or soreness. It fades within twenty-four hours.

(2) A second-degree erythema is a more marked reddening of the skin, with slight irritation. It fades in two or three days.

(3) A third-degree erythema is a marked reddening of the skin, which is hot, sore and œdematous. The redness does not completely disappear on pressure, and the reaction lasts for about a week.

(4) A fourth-degree erythema is similar to a third-degree reaction, except that blisters form.

THICKENING OF THE EPIDERMIS. Damage to the superficial cells is followed by increased reproduction of those in the stratum germinativum. This leads to thickening of the epidermis, which acts as a protection against the rays, so that stronger doses are required to repeat an erythema reaction.

DESQUAMATION. This occurs after the erythema has subsided and is the casting off of dead cells from the surface of the body. It is an acceleration of a normal process and the acceleration is due to the damage to the cells caused by the ultra-violet rays. The amount of peeling varies with the strength of the erythema reaction. After a first-degree erythema the increase in desquamation is imperceptible, after a second-degree erythema there is fine, powdery peeling, while after a third- or fourth-degree erythema there is free peeling. The peeling tends to reduce the resistance gained by the thickening of the epidermis.

PIGMENTATION. Rays with wave-lengths between 2,900 and 3,300 Å are absorbed in the deep epidermis and initiate a chemical action which results in the conversion of the amino acid tyrosine into the pigment melanin. The extent of the pigmentation varies in different individuals, being more marked in those with dark than with fair complexions, and the colour varies somewhat with rays from different sources. That produced by the sun or carbon arc is brown, while that which follows exposure to a mercury vapour lamp is greyish in colour. The pigmentation appears to act as a protection against carcinoma of the skin, which may follow repeated and prolonged exposure of a lightly pigmented skin to ultra-violet rays. It is thought by some authorities to increase the resistance of the skin to infection.

EFFECTS OF ABIOTIC RAYS. The ultra-violet rays with wave-lengths of less than 2,900 Å are termed abiotic rays, because they are inimical to life. E. H. and W. K. Russell have shown that they inhibit the growth of seedlings and they may kill bacteria on the surface of the skin, although a considerable exposure would be necessary to achieve this effect. As they are absorbed in the superficial epidermis these rays do not affect the underlying tissues, but they may cause damage to superficial cells, particularly the newly formed tissue of a healing wound. The longer rays, with wave-lengths above 2,900 Å, are called biotic rays and are beneficial to life.

Provided that an extensive area of skin is irradiated the following *general effects* are produced:

FORMATION OF VITAMIN D. Ultra-violet rays with wave-lengths between 2,700 and 3,100 Å cause a chemical reaction which results in the conversion of 7-dehydrocholesterol into vitamin D. The 7-dehydrocholesterol is one of the constituents of sebum, and the action takes place on the surface of the skin, or in the superficial layers which have absorbed the sebum, as the rays which produce this effect do not penetrate to the sebaceous glands. Vitamin D is necessary for normal calcium and phosphorous metabolism, as it promotes the absorption of these subtances from the intestine.

ESOPHYLACTIC EFFECT. The reticulo-endothelial system

plays an important part in the body's defence against infection. The cells of the reticulo-endothelial system ingest bacteria and produce antibodies, the stimulus necessary to cause this reaction being the presence of bacteria and their toxins. Some of the reticulo-endothelial cells are situated in the superficial tissues, and so can be affected by ultra-violet rays. The effect of strong doses of ultra-violet rays is to lower the threshold of irritability of the cells, so that antibodies are produced more readily in response to the presence of bacteria and their toxins. Thus the body's resistance to infection is increased, this being known as the esophylactic effect. To produce this effect it is necessary to use rays which penetrate to the levels at which the reticulo-endothelial cells are found, *i.e.* at least as far as the deeper layers of the epidermis. So rays with wave-lengths of more than 2,900 Å must be used.

General Tonic Effect. It is claimed that general ultra-violet irradiation has a general tonic effect, appetite and sleep being improved, nervousness and irritability reduced. There is no definite evidence of this effect, and considerable difference of opinion about it.

Therapeutic Effects of General Ultra-violet Irradiation

There is at present much variety of opinion concerning the therapeutic value of general ultra-violet irradiation, but the treatment may be of value in producing the effects mentioned below:

Formation of Vitamin D. This should be beneficial for rickets and other vitamin D deficiencies, being of use both for the prevention and for the treatment of these conditions. The use of ultra-violet irradiation for this purpose is criticised on the grounds that it is simpler to administer a vitamin D preparation by mouth.

To stimulate the formation of vitamin D a large area of skin must be irradiated, and a prolonged course of treatment is necessary. The source of rays is important. It should give an adequate number of the antirachitic rays (2,700-3,100 Å), but, if possible, none of the shorter band of erythema producing rays (2,500 Å). The latter produce an erythema reaction with a short exposure and, as the dose is judged by the erythema reaction, limit the time for which the treatment is applied. If the treatment is of short duration the patient does not receive enough of the longer, vitamin D producing rays to be effective.

IMPROVED RESISTANCE TO INFECTION. The principle of the esophylactic effect is explained in the section on physiological effects. There is conflicting evidence regarding the value of ultra-violet irradiation for increasing the resistance of the body to infection. Experiments carried out on groups of industrial workers some years ago indicated that no benefit was derived from the treatment. The source of rays used for the experiments was, however, one giving a large proportion of the shorter band of erythema producing rays. Consequently the doses were limited to the time necessary for these rays to produce an erythema reaction, and it is unlikely that the number of the longer, more penetrating rays that were absorbed was sufficient to be effective.

The effect may be utilised as a prophylactic measure against winter colds, etc., and in the treatment of boils and other bacterial infections. The source of rays should be one which gives mainly the longer ultra-violet rays, and a definite erythema reaction should be obtained. A fractional method of irradiation may be used, a strong first-degree dose being given to one-sixth of the body surface at each attendance. A stronger dose can be safely applied to this limited area than is advisable if a larger surface is irradiated.

PIGMENTATION AND IMPROVED CONDITION OF THE SKIN. Certain skin conditions, particularly psoriasis, appear to benefit from general ultra-violet irradiation, but as the etiology of some of these conditions is obscure, it is difficult to explain the beneficial effects. They may be associated with the increased blood supply to the skin, and often the results are most satisfactory when a good pigmentation is obtained. The treatment is most effective, especially for psoriasis, if the source of rays is one which gives mainly the longer ultra-violet rays.

GENERAL TONIC EFFECT. Beneficial effects appear to be obtained in the treatment of patients suffering from debility, children who are underweight, etc. It is, however, difficult to explain these effects or to obtain definite evidence of them.

Therapeutic Effects of Local Ultra-violet Irradiation

INCREASED BLOOD SUPPLY TO THE SKIN. There is dilatation of the blood vessels in the skin, with an increased flow of blood to the area. More oxygen and foodstuffs are made available and the nutrition of the tissues is improved. This effect may be utilised in the treatment of bedsores and other indolent wounds, for certain skin conditions, such as psoriasis, acne and alopecia, and for some superficial circulatory defects, such as chilblains. A second-degree or third-degree erythema dose is given, depending on the size of the area.

DESTRUCTION OF BACTERIA. The erythema produced by local ultra-violet irradiation is essentially an inflammatory reaction. The increased blood supply increases the number of white blood cells and antibodies in the area, and there is exudation of fluid into the tissues from the dilated capillaries. These changes reinforce the body's normal mechanism for destroying bacteria, and the treatment may be used for super-ficial bacterial infections such as boils, infected wounds, adenitis and acne.

A strong inflammatory reaction is desirable, and for an infected wound at least a fourth-degree erythema dose is used. If the area is localised but covered by skin, as in a boil, the exposure is limited to a third-degree erythema dose in order to avoid blistering, while if the condition is widespread, as in acne, a second-degree erythema is used.

In addition to the above mechanism, bacteria on the surface of the body may be destroyed by the direct action of the abiotic rays. This may be of value for infected wounds, but at least a fourth-degree erythema dose must be applied.

DESTRUCTION OF TISSUE. Strong doses of ultra-violet rays may damage or destroy the superficial cells, although it is unlikely that extensive destructive effects can be obtained. The rays may be applied to indolent wounds for this purpose. The short ultra-violet rays are the most effective and a fourth-degree erythema dose or more is required.

STIMULATION OF GROWTH OF EPIDERMIS. Ultra-violet irradiation is followed by thickening of the epidermis, and it has been shown that, following damage to cells by ultra-violet rays, a "repair hormone" is produced. This stimulates the growth of new tissue, so accelerating the healing processes, and will be liberated following the strong doses mentioned above for indolent wounds. The hormone is soluble in water, but not in oil, so a dry or oily dressing should be applied after irradiation.

INCREASED RESISTANCE OF THE SKIN TO INFECTION. This is a result of the increased blood supply and nutrition of the skin, the increased number of white blood cells, and possibly also of the pigmentation. It may be used for preventing the spread of infections, such as boils and acne, a second-degree or third-degree erythema dose being given.

DESQUAMATION. This is of value in the treatment of some skin conditions, particularly acne. In acne there is thickening of the epidermis, the openings of the hair follicles are narrowed and the sebum cannot escape. Peeling results in removal of the thickened layer of epidermis and escape of the contents of the hair follicles. The treatment does not effect a permanent cure, but improves the appearance of the skin and helps to limit the scarring that is liable to occur. The free peeling that follows a third-degree erythema is most effective, but it is often necessary to limit the dose to a second-degree erythema. Acne frequently affects the face, and a third-degree erythema reaction on this area is too painful and unsightly for the majority of patients.

COUNTER-IRRITATION. Absorption of ultra-violet rays is followed by irritation of the superficial sensory nerve endings, and so relief of pain by counter-irritation. A third-degree erythema reaction is the most satisfactory for this purpose, the

M

Kromayer lamp being used if the lesion is very localised, or patches up to 35 square inches treated with the air-cooled lamp. Fourth-degree erythema doses are sometimes used, but if blistering occurs there is danger of infection. Second-degree erythema doses may be used over large areas but are less satisfactory than stronger applications. Ultra-violet irradiation has the advantage over other methods of counter-irritation that the effect is maintained for several days. The treatment may be used for many chronic inflammatory lesions and for the after-effects of trauma. It can be applied to areas where defective skin sensation renders heat treatments unsafe, although its efficacy will be reduced if the skin is insensitive.

Sensitisers

Under certain circumstances an individual may become more susceptible than normal to the effects of some agent, and any factor which increases the sensitivity in this way is termed a sensitiser. There are various agents which act as sensitisers to ultra-violet rays.

The coal tar ointment which is often applied to patches of psoriasis before irradiation is a sensitiser. This is an example of the intentional use of a sensitiser in order to increase the reaction to ultra-violet rays.

Infra-red irradiation immediately before exposure to ultra-violet rays acts as a sensitiser, provided that the erythema caused by the infra-red rays is still present when the ultra-violet rays are applied. The effect may be utilised when a sensitiser is required, but must also be taken into consideration when arranging the treatment of a patient who is receiving irradiation with both types of ray.

Certain drugs act as sensitisers to ultra-violet rays, examples being gold, the sulphonamides, insulin, thyroid extract, quinine and various drugs which have recently become available, such as those of the Tetracycline group. Irradiation of individuals who are taking these drugs may result in excessive erythema reaction or a rash may be produced, the latter being particularly liable to occur in association with gold injections. Great care should be exercised in irradiating a patient who is taking any drug of which the effects, when used in conjunction with ultra-violet rays, have not been fully investigated.

Certain foods may act as sensitisers to ultra-violet rays, examples being strawberries, eggs and lobster.

Some local applications, such as the aniline dyes, are said to increase the sensitivity of the skin to ultra-violet rays.

Contraindications

INDIVIDUALS. Some individuals are unsuitable for treatment with ultra-violet rays.

A very sensitive skin, which reacts strongly and develops little or no resistance, contraindicates both local and general treatment.

General ultra-violet irradiation does not appear to suit some individuals, who develop headache, nausea and possibly vomiting and rise of temperature following exposure. Similar symptoms can be caused by exposure of the back of the head and neck to infra-red rays in the course of the irradiation, in which case their occurrence is prevented by shielding these areas during treatment. If relief cannot be obtained in this way the individual is unsuitable for general irradiation.

TREATMENTS. Ultra-violet irradiation should not be used in conjunction with certain other treatments.

When a patient is taking any of the drugs mentioned above as sensitisers to ultra-violet rays, irradiation with these rays is contraindicated.

Local irradiation with ultra-violet rays should not be applied to an area which has recently been subjected to doses of X-rays. X-rays have a devitalising effect on the tissues and it is possible that ultra-violet irradiation under these conditions may cause carcinoma of the skin. Also, if ultra-violet rays are applied shortly after X-ray therapy, before the reaction to the latter has appeared, the effects of the X-rays are reduced. Three months should elapse after X-ray therapy before ultra-violet irradiation is used on the same area.

DISEASES. Certain diseases contraindicate the use of ultra-violet rays.

Pulmonary tuberculosis is a contraindication to general ultra-violet irradiation and to irradiation of the thorax, as the activity of the disease may be increased.

Acute eczema or dermatitis may be aggravated by ultra-violet irradiation.

Rise in temperature from any cause is a contraindication to general irradiation.

25

TECHNIQUE FOR ULTRA-VIOLET IRRADIATION

Assessment of Doses

THE only satisfactory method of assessing doses of ultra-violet rays is by the erythema reaction.

DEGREES OF ERYTHEMA. The four degrees of erythema have been described. A first-degree erythema is recognised by slight reddening of the skin, which fades within twenty-four hours. A second-degree erythema shows a more marked reddening of the skin, and does not fade so soon. A third-degree erythema is characterised by œdema of the skin, and by intense redness, which does not completely disappear on pressure, a fourth-degree erythema by blister formation. A suberythemal dose is an exposure which produces no visible reaction. The term fifth-degree erythema is sometimes used to denote a dose of double that which is required to produce a fourth-degree erythema. The reaction has the same characteristics as the fourth-degree erythema, but to a more marked extent.

The following factors determine the intensity of the reaction:

(1) THE ARC LAMP. The output of rays varies according to the type of lamp, and may also vary with different lamps of the same type. Each new lamp is tested and the average dose required to produce a certain reaction recorded, usually the exposure needed to obtain a first-degree erythema at 3 feet from the lamp. The output of rays, particularly from a mercury vapour lamp, is liable to be reduced as the lamp ages, and although this is counteracted by reduction of the stabilising resistance, the lamp should be tested at regular intervals to ensure that there is no change in the dose required. It is advisable to use the same lamp throughout a course of treat-

ment, as slight differences may exist between lamps which apparently have the same output.

(2) THE DURATION OF THE EXPOSURE. The longer the exposure the stronger is the reaction produced. If the dose required to produce a first-degree erythema is known, those necessary to produce the other degrees of erythema can be calculated.

A second-degree erythema requires $2\frac{1}{2}$ times the exposure necessary to produce a first-degree erythema.

A third-degree erythema requires 5 times the exposure necessary to produce a first-degree erythema.

A fourth-degree erythema requires 10 times the exposure necessary to produce a first-degree erythema.

A so-called fifth-degree erythema requires 20 times the exposure necessary to produce a first-degree erythema.

A suberythemal dose may be taken as half or two-thirds of that required to produce a first-degree erythema.

(3) PREVIOUS EXPOSURE OF THE AREA. An exposure to ultra-violet rays should not be repeated until the erythema caused by a previous dose has faded, as until this occurs the sensitivity is increased. When the reaction has faded there is thickening of the epidermis, and while this lasts it is necessary to increase the exposure in order to repeat the reaction on the same area of skin. The following increases are necessary:

To repeat a first-degree erythema, 25 per cent. of the previous dose is added.

To repeat a second-degree erythema, 50 per cent. of the previous dose is added.

To repeat a third-degree erythema, 75 per cent. of the previous dose is added.

To repeat a fourth-degree erythema 100 per cent. of the previous dose is added.

A suberythemal dose is increased by about $12\frac{1}{2}$ per cent. of the previous exposure, or a 25 per cent. increase may be made at alternate treatments.

Opinions differ regarding the effect of desquamation on the resistance of the skin, but it has been the writer's experience when treating patients with arc lamps that once free peeling has taken place the increased resistance is lost, and the dose should be reduced to that given at the first attendance. Also that fine peeling causes a slight reduction in the resistance, and if this occurs the reaction can be repeated without increasing the exposure. This is, of course, subject to variation in individual patients, and the situation may be different following exposure to natural sunlight. After a first-degree erythema reaction or a suberythemal dose there is no visible peeling, but it is assumed that imperceptible peeling takes place within three weeks, and after an interval in treatment of this duration the dose should be reduced to that given at the first attendance. If the interval is more than 10 days, but less than three weeks, no increase in the dose is made.

(4) DISTANCE BETWEEN THE LAMP AND THE PATIENT. The rays emitted from the majority of ultra-violet lamps obey the law of inverse squares, so the intensity of rays varies inversely with the square of the distance from the burner. Thus the intensity of the radiation at 1 foot is 4 times that at 2 feet and 9 times that at 3 feet. This must be taken into account when calculating doses. If 4 minutes at 3 feet are required to produce a certain reaction, and the exposure is to be given at 18 inches, as the distance is halved, the duration must be divided by 4, *i.e.* 2^2, and 1 minute is required. The following formula may be used to calculate doses at different distances from the lamp:

$$\text{New dose} = \frac{\text{Old dose} \times \text{New distance}^2}{\text{Old distance}^2}$$

(5) THE ANGLE AT WHICH THE RAYS STRIKE THE SKIN. In accordance with the cosine law, maximum absorption takes place when the rays strike the skin at a right angle. If this does not occur, the intensity of the reaction is reduced.

(6) THE SENSITIVENESS OF THE PATIENT. The reaction of different individuals to ultra-violet irradiation varies considerably, fair and auburn haired people often being more sensitive than those of darker complexion. Sensitivity does not always correspond to the colouring, and each patient should be asked whether he reacts strongly to sunlight.

Small children do not readily show an erythema reaction, and excess treatment is most often indicated by general symptoms such as irritability and vomiting. Satisfactory dosage results in increased appetite and weight, and the child becomes placid and sleeps well. Children under 2 years of age should receive half the adult dose, those between 2 and 6 two-thirds of this dose.

The sensitivity of the skin varies in different parts of the body. Exposed surfaces are less sensitive than those which are normally covered by clothing, and the extensor surfaces are less sensitive than the flexor aspects. The dorsum of the hand requires about 5 times the normal dose, the palm of the hand 15, and the sole of the foot 25 times this dose. Mucous membranes need about twice as long an exposure as the skin.

If the patient is taking any of the sensitisers considered in the previous chapter, the reaction is liable to be increased.

Infra-red irradiation applied immediately before exposure to ultra-violet rays increases the reaction, but if applied after the ultra-violet irradiation, before the erythema from the latter appears, it reduces the effects. Simultaneous irradiation with both types of ray does not affect the reaction.

Because so many factors affect the sensitiveness of the patient, test doses should commonly be carried out before commencing a course of treatment. There are, however, a few occasions on which the test dose provides little useful information and may be omitted, for instance, when treating an area devoid of skin.

Test Doses

Test doses are used to determine either the output of a lamp or the sensitivity of a patient.

TECHNIQUE. The same basic technique is used whatever the purpose of the test dose. A suitable area of skin is chosen, cleaned with ether soap and water, then dried. Three holes, usually of different shapes, are cut in a piece of thick paper which is placed over the area and secured with adhesive plaster so that it lies flat on the skin. The holes should be close together, or there may be slight differences in their distances from the lamp or in the angle at which the rays strike the skin. The surrounding skin is protected, and the areas covered while the lamp is arranged in position. The centre area is exposed for the time that is expected to produce the required reaction, one of the others for a slightly shorter, the other for a slightly longer period. The intervals depend on the dose used. If it were anticipated that the required reaction would be produced in two minutes, the areas would be exposed for one and a half, two, and two and a half minutes respectively; but if it were anticipated that six minutes would be required, doses of five, six and seven minutes would be used. Considering the former example, all three areas are exposed for one and a half minutes, then one area covered and the other two exposed for the next half minute. Finally, a second area is covered and the remaining one exposed for a further half minute. The areas are examined an appropriate time after the exposure, to ascertain which shows the required reaction.

OUTPUT OF A LAMP. It is necessary to test the output of every new lamp, and all lamps should be tested at intervals to ensure that there is no change in their output.

The object of the test is to ascertain the average dose required to produce a certain reaction, usually a first-degree erythema at 3 feet, so the test should be carried out on several individuals of average sensitivity. The area of skin selected should be one usually covered by clothing, which has not recently been exposed to the sun or other sources of ultra-violet rays. The abdomen is a suitable area. Each of the three areas exposed should be about one square inch in size. When the doses required on the different individuals have been determined, the average is taken as the standard dose for that particular lamp.

SENSITIVITY OF THE PATIENT. In most cases a test dose should precede a course of treatment by ultra-violet rays, in order to determine the dose required to produce the desired reaction on the particular patient.

When the test dose precedes general irradiation, fairly large areas (*e.g.* 2 square inches) should be exposed. The abdomen is the most satisfactory area on which to carry out the test, as the skin is more sensitive than that of other parts of the body. Washing of the skin does not precede general irradiation and so can be omitted before the test dose.

For a test dose prior to local irradiation, smaller areas may be exposed, *e.g.* half to one square inch. It is most satisfactory to perform the test on the area that is subsequently to be irradiated, as the sensitivity of the skin varies in different parts of the body, and also appears to be influenced by lesions of underlying structures. For example, very large doses are frequently required to obtain a reaction of the skin over an osteo-arthritic joint. The reaction from the test dose will probably still be present when the patient attends for her first treatment, but the areas can be protected with petroleum jelly. If it is inconvenient to apply the test dose to the area which is to be treated, another area of comparable sensitivity may be used. For example, a test dose on the face would give a very unsightly reaction, and before irradiating this area the test may be carried out on the flexor aspect of the forearm, which is of about the same sensitivity.

A first-degree erythema may be used for the test, the dose needed for the desired reaction being calculated from this. A more accurate guide to the required dose is, however, obtained by using the degree of erythema that is subsequently to be applied.

Technique for General Irradiation

CHOICE OF LAMP. If a group of patients is to be irradiated, the Centrosol or the group model of fluorescent tubes is used. For individual treatments the air-cooled mercury vapour lamp or the tunnel model of fluorescent tubes is chosen. The mercury vapour lamps have the disadvantage that the spectrum contains many of the shorter ultra-violet rays, which are undesirable for general treatments. The fluorescent tubes give a satisfactory spectrum.

PREPARATION OF APPARATUS. A mercury vapour lamp is lit five minutes before use to allow the output of rays to reach maximum intensity, and during this time it is placed in such a position that the rays do not shine on those in the room. The fluorescent tubes require no special preparation, but when using the tunnel model it is necessary to check that the plinth is in the correct position below the centre of the lamp.

PREPARATION OF PATIENT. The patient is asked whether he is hypersensitive to sunlight, and his case papers examined to ensure that he is not taking any drug that would act as a sensitiser. He is warned of the expected reaction, and asked to look for an erythema four to twelve hours later and to report on this and any other effects that he may have noticed. A test dose should precede the treatment, and the subsequent dose is arranged according to the result.

In order that the maximum area of skin shall be irradiated the patient wears only a slip, and it is important that the same area of skin is exposed on each occasion. Irradiation of an area which had been covered on previous occasions, and so had not developed resistance, would result in a very uncomfortable reaction. The eyes of the operator and patient must be protected from the rays. The operator usually wears goggles with Chance's Crookes A lenses or some other filter which absorbs ultra-violet rays. The goggles must be covered in at the sides and fit closely round the eyes. The patient may wear goggles also, but in hospital practice each patient is often given a shade made of two layers of thick paper and fixed in position with a bandage tied round the forehead. This shade must extend well beyond the eyes. If infants object to a shade or goggles, a screen may be held between the face and the lamp. The patient is warned of the effects of the rays on the eyes.

ARRANGEMENT OF LAMP AND PATIENT. The distance must be correct and exact. When the Centrosol lamp is used a circle is usually painted on the floor with a radius of 3 feet from the lamp, and the patients sit on chairs round this circle, The operator should see that the patients are sitting so that the part to be irradiated is above this line and that the centre of the arc is opposite the middle of the body—that is, the lower end of the sternum, or the middle of the back. The lamp must be turned on five minutes before commencing treatment, so either the lamp or the patients must be covered while they are being arranged in position.

If the group model of fluorescent tubes is used the patients are usually treated when standing, in order that as large an area of skin as possible may be irradiated, and full use made of the 4-foot tubes. Special rests are made to support the patients during treatment, and the standing position should not be used without these. Standing for some time with no support, and possibly with the eyes covered, is very fatiguing, especially for debilitated patients. A circle can be painted on the floor, as for the Centrosol lamp. The patients are arranged in position before the lamp is turned on, no warming up time being necessary.

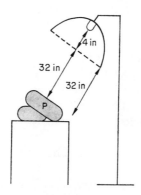

FIG. 199.—ARRANGEMENT OF AIR-COOLED MERCURY VAPOUR
LAMP.

If an air-cooled mercury vapour lamp is used, the patient is generally treated in oblique side lying. He is arranged in position, fully supported with pillows, and covered while the position of the lamp is adjusted. The lamp is arranged so that the rays strike the skin at right angles and the arc tube is opposite to the centre of the body, *i.e.* a point midway between the 7th cervical vertebra and the knee joints. The distance from the burner to the patient must be measured accurately. It is not wise to measure from the burner while the lamp is on, so the distance from the burner to some point on the reflector should be determined while the lamp is cold. Measurements are subsequently taken from this point, allowance being made for the extra inches from the burner. In Fig. 199 the burner lies 4 inches back from the opening of the reflector. Distances are measured from the rim of the reflector, allowing for these 4 inches.

If the tunnel model of fluorescent tubes is used, the patient lies either prone or supine under the centre of the lamp, which is lowered to the level at which the tubes are 18 inches from the patient.

Before commencing treatment the patient is warned not to move from position or touch the lamp.

THE TREATMENT. The fluorescent tubes are turned on or, if the mercury vapour lamp is used, the patient is uncovered. The time is kept accurately either with an alarm clock or else with the second hand of a watch. Where there are several patients sitting round a lamp for group treatment, each requiring a different dose, a list of the times must be kept and each one informed when to turn and expose the other side of the body, and when to come away from the lamp. The patient should be assisted in turning or leaving the lamp, to ensure that he does not approach too close to it as he moves.

When using the tunnel model of fluorescent tubes, an active patient may turn over with the tunnel in position, provided that the physiotherapist supervises the procedure. With less active patients and when using the mercury vapour lamp for individual treatments, the lamp is removed while the patient turns over. Then, with the patient covered, the position and distance of the lamp are checked before continuing the exposure.

During the treatment the operator ensures that the patients do not alter their positions and, if the treatment is being given in sitting, that they sit up straight. She must also ensure that the patients do not remove their goggles or shades. These points are particularly important when treating children.

At the end of the treatment the lamp is switched off or removed. The mercury vapour lamp should not be turned off if required for other patients, as the arc will not strike while the lamp is hot.

RECORDS OF TREATMENT. Notes should be kept of the date, lamp used, part exposed, time of exposure, distance of patient from lamp, effects of rays, including erythema reaction, and other good or ill effects. The patient should be weighed weekly, as persistent loss of weight may indicate unsuitability for this form of treatment.

DOSAGE. For general irradiation of the body, the aim is commonly to produce a first-degree erythema reaction. Suberythemal doses are used for cases where ultra-violet rays must be given very cautiously, as in certain cases of tuberculosis where the lungs show signs of the disease, or debility after illnesses or associated with old age, or if a prolonged course of treatment is considered desirable.

Usually the whole body is irradiated at each attendance, the anterior and posterior aspects being exposed. Some authorities advise that only the back of the trunk and legs should be irradiated on the first occasion, then the front of the same areas, to ensure that there are no adverse general effects, before proceeding to the full treatment. A fractional method may be used and for this the body is divided into four or six areas—the front and back of the trunk, the front and back of the legs, and possibly the sides of the body. This method is often used when the esophylactic effect is required, it is useful if only a small lamp is available or if the patient is tall, and it is sometimes used in the treatment of generalised skin conditions, such as psoriasis, when a second-degree erythema dose may be given to one area at each attendance. When using first-degree or suberythemal doses one or more areas may be irradiated at each attendance. Sometimes the patient attends three times a week, one area being irradiated each time. Thus each area is treated once a fortnight, and no increase of dose is necessary.

PROGRESSION OF DOSES. An increase in the dose is necessary if the erythema reaction is to be repeated, but the patient should be questioned before deciding each dose. The usual increase may not be given on account of an excessive reaction or ill effects from the previous dose, or because there was an interval of ten days or more between irradiations. A first-degree erythema dose is commonly increased by 25 per cent. and a suberythemal dose by $12\frac{1}{2}$ per cent. of the previous exposure, and in most cases this increase is satisfactory at the beginning of a course. It is, however, not uncommon to find that as the dose becomes longer it is sufficient to increase by a smaller proportion of the previous exposure.

FREQUENCY OF IRRADIATION. First-degree erythema doses are usually given on alternate days, as this allows time for fading of the reaction resulting from the previous exposure, although if a fractional method is used the patient can attend daily, different areas being exposed on consecutive days. Sub-erythemal doses can be applied daily.

Technique for Local Irradiation

CHOICE OF LAMP. The two lamps commonly used for local irradiation are the air-cooled mercury vapour lamp and the Kromayer lamp. The former is used if a fairly large area is to be irradiated, the latter if the area is small or if it is desirable to use one of the special applicators. Both these lamps give a large proportion of the short ultra-violet rays, and filters may be used to absorb these, for example, a blue uviol filter, Cellophane, liquid paraffin or cod liver oil.

PREPARATION OF LAMP. A mercury vapour lamp is lighted five minutes before the irradiation, and if the Kromayer lamp is used the water must be circulating before the arc is struck. The window of the Kromayer lamp is cleaned with methylated ether before commencing treatment.

PREPARATION OF THE PATIENT. As a rule the skin is washed with soap and water before a local exposure, and, if it is greasy, ether soap should be used. Sometimes special preparation of the area is required. For example, liquid paraffin is used in some cases of psoriasis, and special methods are necessary if the area is not covered by skin. These are considered with the treatment of wounds. The patient is supported in a comfortable position, so that he will not move during the treatment, and the part round the area to be irradiated is protected. A sheet of thick paper with a hole in the centre can be used, or towels may be arranged round the area. If the part has been treated previously, care must be taken to expose exactly the same area of skin at each attendance. The eyes must be protected with goggles or a shade.

Before commencing treatment the patient should receive the same warnings as those which precede a general treatment. He should also be warned of the erythema reaction and subsequent pigmentation.

ARRANGEMENT OF THE LAMP AND PATIENT. If the air-cooled mercury vapour lamp is used, the skin is covered while the lamp is brought into position and arranged so that the rays strike the skin at right angles. The distance is measured as for general treatments.

The Kromayer lamp may be used at a few inches from the skin (usually 2 or 4), in contact or with various applicators. The lamp is held in position by the operator, and so both she and the patient must be adequately supported. It is difficult to hold the lamp steady in the correct position, and so, unless the dose is very brief and given in contact, the lamp should be supported, possibly on pillows. When the treatment is to be given with the lamp at 2 or 4 inches, the eyes of the patient and operator must be protected and the area localised. Care must be taken that the rays strike the skin at a right angle and that the distance is correct. It is usually easiest to measure this with a ruler. When the treatment is to be given in contact the exact area to be treated is ascertained and, if necessary, marked. In all cases the protective cap of the lamp is retained in position until the commencement of the treatment. The use of applicators is considered separately.

TREATMENT. The area is uncovered or the protective cap of the Kromayer lamp removed. If the latter is used in contact with the tissues it must be held firmly and steadily against the skin. The dose is timed accurately, the operator ensuring that the patient does not move or remove his goggles or shade.

At the end of the treatment the lamp is removed. If an intense reaction is expected, steps may be taken to protect the area before the patient leaves the department. When a fourth-degree erythema is produced on an area covered by clothes, zinc or boracic ointment should be applied on a piece of lint to protect the blister which will form, from irritation by rubbing of the clothes.

NOTES. These should be kept as for general treatments. Diagrams showing the areas treated on each occasion are frequently of considerable assistance.

DOSAGE. For local irradiation any degree of erythema may be used. A second-degree erythema can be applied to a large area (up to one-sixth of the body surface), but on account of the intense irritation a third-degree should be given only to a smaller area, 35 square inches being the maximum. When a blister is produced the area should be considerably less in extent, not more than the size of the window of the Kromayer lamp, although a fourth-degree erythema dose can be applied to a larger area if it is not covered by skin, *e.g.* to a wound. A fifth-degree erythema dose can be used on a wound, but if applied to the skin the area should not be more than the size of a shilling, as the blistering is more intense than with the fourth-degree reaction.

When considering the dose required the patient's case papers must be examined and enquiries made regarding sensitivity, as before a general treatment. Having calculated the dose that will probably be needed, a test dose is carried out before commencing treatment. If this does not produce the reaction that is required the necessary adjustments are made. For example, 2 minutes at 18 inches might be the average dose for a third-degree erythema, but produce only a second-degree reaction on the patient. Then 4 minutes at 18 inches would be given.

PROGRESSION OF DOSES. It is usually necessary to increase the duration of the exposure in order to repeat a reaction on the same area of skin. This can be calculated as explained on p. 326, always taking into consideration the reaction obtained from the previous exposure and making allowance for any peeling that has taken place. If the area has partly peeled it is wiser to delay treatment until the peeling is complete. Some, but not all, parts of the area have lost their resistance and an uneven reaction would be obtained. A first-degree erythema dose may be given on alternate days, a

N

second-degree erythema dose twice a week and a third-degree erythema dose once a week. Ten to fourteen days should elapse before repeating a fourth-degree erythema dose.

Special Techniques

TREATMENT OF WOUNDS. For these all aseptic precautions must be observed.

Wounds are cleaned in the usual way. Crusts formed on septic wounds should be removed, but the scab which may form over a healing wound is left. After cleansing, the surface is dried, as fluid on the surface would interfere with penetration of the rays. The skin round the wound is protected with sterilised lint or a sterile paper towel, and the area irradiated.

Fourth-degree or fifth-degree erythema doses are used for infected or indolent wounds, in order to provoke a strong inflammatory reaction and possibly to sterilise the wound and destroy superficial tissue, with subsequent liberation of the repair hormone. The irradiation must be confined to the area of the wound, or blistering of the surrounding skin will result. The irradiation is frequently followed by increased discharge. If it is desired to repeat the reaction, no increase in dose is necessary, as there is no skin over the surface of the wound to develop resistance. A first-degree or second-degree erythema dose to the skin surrounding the wound is often used in conjunction with the above treatment. The aims are to increase the blood supply to the area and to increase the resistance of the skin to infection. Progression of doses on this area is necessary, as the skin develops an increased resistance.

When a wound is healing, first-degree or second-degree erythema doses may be given to increase the blood supply and stimulate the growth of epidermis. Care must be taken that the newly formed epithelial tissue is not damaged, and it may be protected with sterile petroleum jelly. The abiotic rays would be harmful, and a filter may be used to eliminate these. The blue uviol filter, Cellophane or sterile oil sprayed over the surface of the wound may be used for this purpose.

TREATMENT OF CAVITIES. Deep wounds, sinuses and

other cavities may be irradiated with a suitable quartz applicator attached to the Kromayer lamp. This necessitates an increase in the exposure, according to the rod used. The applicator must be sterilised before use and this may be done by wrapping it in gauze, to prevent damage, and boiling it for five minutes. The cavity is cleaned in the usual way, the rod introduced, making sure that it reaches to the base of the cavity, and the area irradiated.

TREATMENT WITH COMPRESSION. Local ultra-violet irradiation may be applied with compression in order to eliminate the blood from the area, and so allow a deeper penetration of rays. The rays which penetrate more deeply are those with wave-lengths of more than 3,300 Å, which are normally absorbed by the blood in the superficial capillaries. The method has been used mainly in the treatment of lupus vulgaris, in order to allow the rays to penetrate to the site of the lesion, which is in the dermis. Ultra-violet irradiation is rarely used for this condition nowadays, but may occasionally be employed when other forms of treatment are contra-indicated, and compression may be applied for the treatment of other conditions. When applying the treatment with compression, a convex quartz applicator is attached to the Kromayer lamp, thus enabling even pressure to be applied to the area. The patient and operator must both be fully supported, and counterpressure applied on the opposite aspect of the part being treated.

Dangers and Precautions

(1) CONJUNCTIVITIS. Exposure of the eyes to ultra-violet rays causes conjunctivitis. The onset is delayed for some time after the irradiation, and the symptoms are pain, a "gritty" feeling in the eyes, photophobia and lacrimation. Fortunately, the symptoms commonly clear up in a few days, leaving no ill effects, although after one attack the individual is more sensitive on subsequent occasions. The treatment of mild cases is to bathe the eyes with boracic lotion, or use drops of liquid paraffin or castor oil. In more severe cases dark glasses should

be worn, and in some cases it may be necessary to remain in a dark room for a day or two.

To prevent the occurrence of conjunctivitis, protective shades or goggles must be worn by the patient and operator, patients must be warned of the danger to the eyes, and children wearing shades must be closely watched, as they are liable to push the shade on one side and look at the lamp. Lamps must be arranged so that the rays do not shine on other people in the department.

(2) OVERDOSE. The skin becomes red, hot, and extremely sore, and if the overdose is severe there may be blister formation. General symptoms may occur if a large area of skin is affected and include headache, vomiting, a high temperature, and collapse.

The precautions against an overdose lie in careful technique.

The strength of the rays from the lamp must be known, and the same lamp should be used throughout the course.

Before treatment is commenced, enquiries must be made to ensure that the patient is not hypersensitive to sunlight, and test doses are used to ascertain the initial dose required for each patient. Progression of doses must be made with care, considering the reaction to the previous treatment and the time that has elapsed since the last exposure. The same area of skin must be exposed each time a treatment is repeated on the same part.

Patients must be warned not to move after they have been arranged in position. The distance of the patient from the arc should be carefully measured, and the lamp arranged so that the rays strike the skin at a right angle.

The exposure must be timed carefully and notes made for each patient.

If a patient does receive an overdose, infra-red rays should be applied immediately to the area which has been irradiated with ultra-violet rays. The exposure should cause an infra-red ray erythema over the whole area. The production of an infra-red ray erythema diminishes the intensity of the ultra-violet ray erythema which will appear later. When the patient arrives home he should apply cold cream to the part. Later, if there is much irritation, calamine lotion can be used.

(3) ELECTRIC SHOCK. This might occur as a result of touching some exposed part of the circuit, or, if the live wire of the supply came in contact with the casing of the lamp, which was not earthed, any person touching the casing while connected to earth would receive an earth shock. The necessary precautions are considered in Chapter 12.

(4) BURNS. Heat burns could occur from touching a hot part of the lamp, or from hot quartz if the burner were to burst when placed over the patient, although this is a rare occurrence.

The patient must be warned not to touch the lamp, and it is safer never to put a mercury vapour burner over a patient.

(5) CHILL. The patient receiving general treatment may catch a chill if the room is too cold, or if there is a draught. The mercury vapour lamps and fluorescent tubes do not give many infra-red rays, and the patient may become cold during treatment. To avoid this, infra-red irradiation may be given at the same time as the ultra-violet irradiation. Simultaneous irradiation with infra-red and ultra-violet rays does not affect the reaction to the latter.

(6) CONTRAINDICATIONS. The conditions in which ultra-violet irradiation is contraindicated are considered on pp. 323 and 324.

26

ULTRA-SONIC THERAPY

Ultra-sonic Energy

NATURE OF ULTRA-SONIC WAVES. Sound waves are longitudinal waves in matter and consist of a to and fro movement of particles in the direction in which the rays are travelling. They differ from electromagnetic waves in that the latter consist of an up and down movement of the ether and can be transmitted through space, whereas the sound waves consist of a to and fro movement of particles and require some material medium through which to travel. The medium must have some degree of elasticity in order that the particles shall resist deformation and then rebound to maintain the to and fro movement. As the particles move to and fro, areas of compression alternate with areas of rarefaction.

The human ear can detect sound waves with frequencies of between 30 and 20,000 cycles per second, but not those of higher frequencies. The latter are ultra-sonic waves. The frequencies of the waves employed for medical purposes are between 500,000 and 3,000,000 cycles per second, that of 1,000,000 cycles per second being the most widely used.

Those properties of ultra-sonic waves which are relevant to physiotherapy are considered below.

FREQUENCY, VELOCITY AND WAVE-LENGTH. The waves are produced by vibration of matter and have the same frequency as the vibrations which set them up. The frequency of any particular wave is constant, but the velocity varies in different media being, for example, greater in water than in air. Velocity is equal to the product of frequency and wave-length, so the wave-length also varies in different media, and the waves must be defined according to their frequency.

TRANSMISSION BY DIFFERENT MEDIA. The waves travel more easily in some media than in others, depending on the ease and speed with which the material can be deformed. This is indicated by the *characteristic acoustic impedance* of the material. The waves travel more easily through a medium with a high than with a low characteristic acoustic impedance. They pass easily through steel, in which it is high, rather less so through water and with difficulty through air, of which the characteristic acoustic impedance is low.

When a wave encounters a different medium from that in which it has been travelling, it may be reflected, transmitted or absorbed.

REFLECTION. The wave is turned back from the surface of the new medium and the angle of reflection is equal to the angle of incidence. The proportion of rays reflected depends on the characteristic acoustic impedances of the materials concerned. Those of which it is low tend to reflect the rays, and the greater the difference in the characteristic acoustic impedances of the media, the greater is the proportion of rays reflected.

TRANSMISSION. The wave may continue to travel through the new medium. If it strikes the surface at a right angle it continues to travel in the same straight line, but otherwise *refraction* occurs. The direction and extent to which the ray bends depends on its relative velocities in the two media. Waves passing from a medium in which the velocity is low, such as air, to one in which it is high, such as water, bend away from the normal (Fig. 200) and vice versa. The greater the difference in velocities, the greater is the angle through which the wave bends.

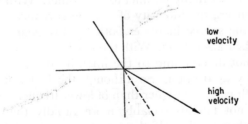

low velocity

high velocity

FIG. 200.—REFRACTION OF ULTRA-SONIC WAVES.

ABSORPTION. As a beam of waves passes through any medium some are absorbed, resulting in reduction in intensity (Fig. 201). The beam is reduced to half its previous intensity

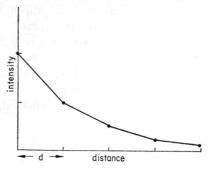

FIG. 201.—REDUCTION IN INTENSITY OF A BEAM OF RAYS.
d = ½ value distance.

in a certain distance, which is termed the *half-value distance* and depends on the nature of the medium and the frequency of the waves. The waves of higher frequencies are absorbed more rapidly than those of lower frequencies, so have a smaller half-value distance. In the tissues of the body, waves with a frequency of 1,000,000 cycles per second have a half-value distance of about 5 centimetres, those of 3,000,000 cycles per second 1·5 centimetres.

DIVERGENCE OF WAVES. Sound waves from a point source diverge and obey the law of inverse squares. As the frequency increases the divergence becomes less and waves with a frequency of 1,000,000 cycles per second, coming from a point source, are virtually parallel to each other. With waves of lower frequencies, the intensity of a beam is reduced as the distance from the source increases both by divergence of the waves and by their absorption. With those of higher frequencies the waves do not diverge and so the intensity of the beam is reduced only by absorption. So although the half-value distance is less with waves of higher than of lower frequencies, the intensity does not fall appreciably more rapidly than with those of lower frequencies. If the waves are emitted from a flat disc, such as the treatment head of the ultra-sonic machine, their distribution is complex, but the same principle applies.

Production of Ultra-sonic Waves

PRINCIPLES OF PRODUCTION. Sound and ultra-sound waves are both produced by the vibration of matter, but no mechanical device can vibrate with a sufficiently high frequency to produce ultra-sonic waves. One method of producing ultra-sonic waves used for therapeutic purposes is by the vibration of a crystal of quartz or some similar material. As explained in the section on interference in Chapter 18, the application of a P.D. across a suitable crystal causes distortion of the crystal, and this is followed by a series of changes in shape, the frequency of which is determined by the way in which the crystal is cut. It is this oscillation of the crystal that sets the particles of matter in motion and produces the ultra-sonic waves (Fig. 202).

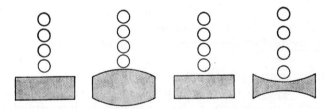

FIG. 202.—PRODUCTION OF ULTRA-SONIC WAVES BY
OSCILLATION OF A QUARTZ CRYSTAL.

THE ULTRA-SONIC GENERATOR. In an ultra-sonic generator a high-frequency alternating current is produced by a valve generator and applied to the crystal, the frequency of the current being the same as the natural frequency of the crystal. In front of the crystal lies a metal diaphragm, which is made to vibrate by the oscillation of the crystal. The ultra-sonic waves are emitted from the diaphragm, which forms the face of the treatment head or transducer.

CONTROL OF OUTPUT. When the machine is turned on the high-frequency current causes oscillation of the crystal. Most machines are constructed so that the frequency of the current is the same as that of the crystal, but some require tuning, on the same principles as the short-wave diathermic machine. The energy applied to the crystal is then increased to the required level. The output is measured in watts per square centimetre of treatment head, a range of from 0·25 to 3 watts per square centimetre being available for treatment purposes. The output is usually assessed by calibrations on the control, although a meter may be used to obtain the correct setting.

Some machines make available a pulsed beam, the output of ultra-sonic waves being intermittent. For example, waves may be emitted for periods of 2 milliseconds, followed by intervals of 8 milliseconds. This gives a pulse ratio of 1 to 5, as the energy is emitted for 2 milliseconds in every 10. The pulse ratio may be varied, perhaps to 1 to 10 and 1 to 20. The advantages of the pulsed beam are considered below.

Physiological and Therapeutic Effects

The waves pass into the tissues in a beam the size of the treatment head, their distribution being complex, but the intensity greatest opposite to the centre of the head. The waves are absorbed by the tissues, so their intensity decreases as the distance from the head increases. The depth of effective penetration depends on the frequency of the waves, and with a frequency of 1,000,000 cycles per second the intensity of waves at a depth of 5 centimetres is approximately half that on the skin.

THERMAL EFFECTS. When the waves are absorbed heat is produced, and this effect is most apparent at the tissue interfaces, as between fat and muscle and at the periosteum.

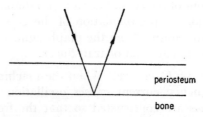

FIG. 203.—REFLECTION OF RAYS BY SURFACE OF NEW MEDIUM.

This is partly due to absorption of the waves when they encounter a new medium and partly to the fact that reflection of the rays by the surface of the new medium results in both the incident and reflected rays passing close together in the old medium. For example, in the periosteum when the rays are reflected by underlying bone (Fig. 203). The heat has similar effects to heat produced in the tissues by other means, so there is increased cell activity and vasodilatation occurs, resulting in an increased blood supply. This makes available more oxygen and foodstuffs, accelerates the removal of waste products and aids the resolution of inflammation.

MECHANICAL EFFECTS. The waves cause a to and fro movement of the particles, and although the actual distance moved by each particle is small, the variations in pressure are considerable and have mechanical effects on the tissues. The permeability of membranes is increased, with consequent acceleration of fluid interchange and absorption. Adherent tissues are loosened, probably due to the separation of collagen fibres from each other and softening of the cement substance. If the movement is excessive there is danger of disruption of the tissues causing cavitation and severe damage, but this should not occur with the intensities used for therapeutic purposes.

There is diversity of opinion regarding the relative value of the thermal and mechanical effects. When a pulsed beam is used the heat is dissipated during the intervals in output, and the thermal effects are minimal, so that the mechanical effects can be obtained without discomfort to the patient. The latter are not affected by the intermittent output, as the variations in pressure are the same as with a continuous beam.

RELIEF OF PAIN. Pain can be relieved by ultra-sonic therapy and, although this may in part be due to the thermal effect, it appears that there is some other mechanism, possibly a direct effect on the nerves, as analgesia can be obtained by the use of a pulsed beam of low intensity, which causes no appreciable heating.

CHEMICAL EFFECTS. It has been shown in the laboratory that ultra-sonic energy can accelerate chemical changes, but there is no evidence of increased chemical reactions in the tissues beyond those which would result from the rise in temperature.

Uses of Ultra-sonic Energy

Ultra-sonic energy has various uses apart from therapy, such as the destruction of tissue and as a diagnostic agent, but these are beyond the scope of this book. It has been used therapeutically for a great variety of conditions and good results reported. In many of these conditions the effects, though beneficial, are not superior to those of other forms of physiotherapy, and the value of ultra-sonic therapy is that it provides an alternative method of treatment. In a few conditions it does appear more effective than other methods.

TRAUMATIC AND INFLAMMATORY CONDITIONS. Ultra-sonic therapy may be used for a variety of traumatic and inflammatory conditions. Following soft tissue injuries the absorption of fluid is promoted and the formation of adhesions reduced, while analgesia permits early use of the part. Care must, however, be taken that further injury is not caused by the injudicious use of exercise in the absence of pain. Increased blood supply should aid tissue repair, and the same effects may be utilised in inflammatory conditions, such as bursitis, capsulitis and tendinitis, the method being particularly indicated when the lesion is at a tissue interface such as a tendon sheath. It is claimed that ultra-sonic therapy is more effective than other methods for heating bones and joints, but it is not certain that this effect is really desirable; in osteo-arthritis and similar conditions heating of the surrounding soft tissues is probably more beneficial. Satisfactory results have, however, been reported in the treatment of ankylosing spondylitis.

SCAR TISSUE. Scar tissue is softened by the application of ultra-sonic waves, and the method is of use both for superficial scars and for more deeply placed fibrous tissue. The latter includes induration following a hæmatoma, carbuncle or similar lesion, also Dupuytren's contracture and plantar fascitis. For softening scar tissue the method appears better than others at present available, although results are not as a rule dramatic.

Dangers and Precautions

There have been alarming reports of the dangers of ultra-sonic therapy, but more recent findings indicate that these are exaggerated and that the treatment is not dangerous provided that certain precautions are observed. The basic condition for the application of a safe treatment is that it should be painless. The principal dangers are:

BURNS. These are heat burns and are due to too great an intensity of radiation. They may occur if excess energy is applied or if the treatment head is allowed to remain stationary during treatment, so that the effects are confined to a small area, also if there is incomplete contact between the treatment head and the tissues, as the energy is then concentrated in the area of contact. This may cause overheating of the tissues or of the transducer, which subsequently burns the patient. Over-heating may result from standing waves set up from superficial bony surfaces, as these surfaces reflect the waves, which pass to and fro between the bone and the treatment head, so that the energy is concentrated in a limited area.

Burns should be avoided so long as the treatment causes no discomfort. Excess sensation of heat should not occur, nor aching, nor pain, either of which is an indication of overheating of the deep tissues. To ensure that the patient can appreciate the degree of heating, the sensation to heat and cold should be tested before the first application, and if it is impaired the treatment should be used only with extreme caution. Superficial bony points should be avoided and the treatment head kept moving and in perfect contact throughout the application. The danger of burns is considerably reduced by the use of a pulsed beam.

Should a burn occur, the procedure is the same as for a short-wave diathermy burn (page 261).

CAVITATION. Excess ultra-sonic energy could disrupt the tissues, but this should not occur so long as the doses do not exceed the suggested level and no discomfort is experienced during treatment.

OVERDOSE. Excess treatment may aggravate symptoms, so doses should be increased cautiously and in accordance with the effects produced.

DAMAGE TO EQUIPMENT. If energy is applied to the crystal with the treatment head in air there is a danger that the waves may be reflected from the air, which is a poor transmitter, back on to the crystal. Waves pass to and fro between the air and the crystal, *i.e.* standing waves are set up, and may increase the vibration of the crystal to such a point that it is shattered.

Contraindications

Ultra-sonic waves should not be applied to specialised tissues such as the eye, ear, ovaries or testes, and some authorities consider that they may have harmful effects on the brain and spinal cord, on sympathetic ganglia and possibly other nerves and on growing ends of bones.

The pregnant uterus should not be treated.

If the blood supply is impaired the dangers are the same as those of other heat treatments, and if ultra-sonic therapy is used under these circumstances the intensity should be kept low.

Ultra-sonic energy should not be applied to a neoplasm, as it may cause metastases, nor where there is active bacterial infection, as spread of infection may result.

Methods of Application

When applying ultra-sonic energy it is essential that the waves are transmitted evenly from the treatment head to the tissues. It is unsatisfactory to attempt transmission through air, as this has a very low characteristic acoustic impedance and so the majority of the waves are reflected by the air away from the patient. Direct application of the transducer to the tissues is also unsatisfactory, as perfect contact is impossible and pockets of air, even those so small as caused by the presence of a hair, result in reflection of the waves and uneven distribution. Consequently some coupling medium must be used. This must be of such a consistency that it makes perfect contact with both the transducer and the tissues, must transmit the waves satisfactorily and have a characteristic acoustic impedance similar to that of steel and the tissues, in order that undue reflection shall not occur. Water is satisfactory, but should be boiled before use to eliminate dissolved gases, which otherwise, under the influence of the waves, form bubbles which collect on immersed objects and interfere with transmission. Various forms of oil and creams can be used, but not all are suitable. Glycerine, liquid paraffin and the contact creams made by manufacturers of the equipment are satisfactory, but the petroleum jelly which has been used in the past, usually mixed with liquid paraffin, gives virtually no transmission. Air bubbles must not be present in the contact medium. The relative merits of application through a contact cream and through water are considered below.

THROUGH CONTACT CREAM OR OIL. This method is satisfactory so long as the surface of the body is sufficiently even for contact between the tissues and the treatment head to be maintained throughout. The skin is smeared liberally with the oil or cream, and the treatment head moved over the area, great care being taken to keep it in perfect contact and in such a position that the beam enters the tissues at right angles to the surface. Deviation from this angle results in refraction of the waves, both at the body surface and as they pass between the different layers of tissue. The velocity of the waves is high in the tissues, so as they enter the body they tend to bend away from the normal and travel parallel to the surface, as in Fig. 200. This limits their depth of penetration. Some physio-therapists find the application easiest with a treatment head that is set straight on the handle, while others prefer one that is placed at an angle. Some transducers are made so that the angle can be adjusted as required.

WATER BATH. This method may be used for parts of the body which are small enough to be immersed in a bath but are too irregular for direct application of the treatment head, also for hypersensitive areas, where contact of the treatment head would cause discomfort. Its disadvantage is that it is not possible to assess the exact amount of energy that is transmitted to the tissues. The treatment head is immersed in the water and moved at a distance of between half and one inch from the part, the surface of the treatment head being kept parallel to that of the skin. If bubbles collect, the treatment should be interrupted while they are wiped from the skin and treatment head.

On the Surface of the Water (Fig. 204). This method may be used where there is some contraindication to immersion of the part in water, but the area is too irregular or sensitive for direct application of the treatment head. The treatment head is placed in the water and a reflector directs the ultra-sonic waves to the surface (Fig. 204). The part is supported so that the skin is just in contact with the water.

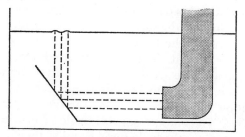

FIG. 204.—USE OF REFLECTOR TO DIRECT WAVES TO THE SURFACE OF THE WATER.

Water Bag. A rubber bag containing boiled water is placed in contact with the skin and the ultra-sonic waves applied through the water, the treatment head being moved over the further surface of the bag.

Technique of Treatment

Preparation of the Apparatus. The machine is tested to ensure that it is working correctly. This can be done by splashing a few drops of water on the surface of the treatment head and turning up the controls. When energy is applied the waves cause vibration of the water, which appears to boil.

Preparation of the Patient. Clothing is removed from the area to be treated and the skin sensation to heat and cold tested before the first application. The part is swabbed with oil or immersed in water and supported comfortably. The patient is warned that he will experience a sensation of warmth and that any discomfort must be reported immediately. It is important that he understands the nature of the treatment and that excess heat may cause a burn.

APPLICATION OF TREATMENT. The treatment head is placed in the water or in contact with the tissues and the output increased to the required level. The treatment head is then moved slowly in relationship to the part, avoiding superficial bony areas and maintaining perfect contact and the correct angle throughout. A circular movement is usually the most satisfactory. Care must be taken when treating thin areas, such as the hand, as waves may be reflected back into the tissues by air on the further surface. At the end of the session the controls are returned to zero and the treatment head removed.

DOSE. For recent injuries and acute conditions it is advisable to commence with a low intensity application of short duration, for example, 0·25 watts per square centimetre for 3 minutes, though the treatment can be applied twice daily. For chronic conditions the initial dose may be $\frac{1}{2}$ watt per square centimetre for 5 minutes, once daily or on alternate days. The depth of the structure should be considered, remembering that the intensity of radiation decreases as the distance from the surface increases. Increases in dose are made at subsequent treatments, in accordance with the effects observed. A sensation of warmth is expected if a continuous beam is used, but aggravation of symptoms indicates excess treatment. The output is usually increased to 1 to 1$\frac{1}{2}$ watts per square centimetre but 2 to 2$\frac{1}{2}$ watts per square centimetre may be required for deeply placed structures and over thick muscle masses. The maximum output that is considered safe for treatment purposes is 3 watts per square centimetre. Ten minutes is usually an adequate duration for treatment of limited areas, fifteen minutes being required for more extensive regions.

27

MICROWAVE DIATHERMY

MICROWAVE diathermy is irradiation of the tissues with the shorter wireless, or Hertzian rays. The rays used are electromagnetic waves with wavelengths between those of infra-red rays and the waves emitted by the short-wave diathermic current. There is some variation in definition, but the waves with wavelengths of between 1 metre and 1 centimetre may be classified as microwaves. They may alternatively be termed decimetre waves. Waves with a wavelength of 12·25 cm. and a frequency of 2,450 megacycles/second are frequently used and some use is made of those with a wavelength of 69 cm., frequently 433·92 megacycles/second.

Production and Application

PRODUCTION OF WAVES. Wireless waves are produced by high-frequency currents and have the same frequency as the currents which produce them. The principles of production of the currents which set up microwaves are similar to those for other high-frequency currents, but in order to obtain the necessary very high frequency a special type of valve, called a magnetron, is used. As with other valves, the magnetron requires time to warm up, so output is not obtained immediately the apparatus is switched on, and a stand-by switch should be provided for use between treatments. This enables the output circuit to be disconnected without cutting off the current to the valves, so that repeated heating and cooling of the valves are avoided.

Current is carried from the high-frequency circuit by a coaxial cable. A coaxial cable consists of a central wire with an outer metal sheath which is separated from the wire by insulating material. The wire and the sheath run parallel to each other throughout and form the output and return wires of the circuit. This construction is necessary for the very high frequency current used, and the cable must be of the correct length for the particular frequency.

The coaxial cable carries the current to a small aerial from which the microwaves are emitted. The aerial is mounted in a reflector, which is packed with some material which transmits the waves, so forming a solid unit. The whole device is used to direct the waves onto the tissues and may be termed the emitter, the director or the applicator. The patient does not form part of the circuit, which is constructed in such a way that no tuning is necessary for individual treatments.

Microwaves can interfere with radio communications so, as with short-wave diathermy, the generator must be constructed so that interference is minimal, and only specified frequencies may be used for medical work. The frequencies of 2,450 megacycles/second and 433·92 megacycles/second, wavelengths 12·25 and 69 cm. respectively, are among those permitted.

APPLICATION TO THE TISSUES. The emitter, as described above, comprises the aerial, reflector and packing, and various types are available. Those most commonly used are placed at a distance from the body and the waves pass through the intervening air to reach the tissues. Emitters of this type may be circular or rectangular in shape. The circular ones give a beam of rays which is circular on cross section and is said to be more dense at the periphery than in the centre (Fig. 205). The rectangular emitter provides a beam which is oval on cross section and is of greatest density centrally (Fig. 205).

In both cases the rays given off from the emitter diverge, so that their density becomes less as the distance from the emitter increases. Reduction in the intensity of the beam is also caused by absorption of the rays. The distance from the skin at which these emitters are used depends on the particular emitter, the output of the generator and the structure to be treated. Commonly it is between 4 and 8 inches. A greater distance is used for large than for small areas, and requires a greater output.

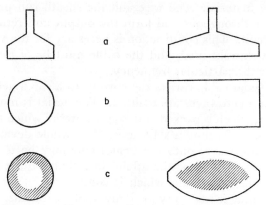

FIG. 205—MICROWAVE DIATHERMY EMITTERS AND DISTRIBUTION OF WAVES.
(a) Side of emitter. (b) Surface of emitter. (c) Distribution of waves.

Small emitters are made for use in contact with the tissues and the treatment of cavities, but do not appear to have been as effective as the distance emitters.

Recently an emitter with a concave surface, which fits round the body, has been used with the longer waves (69 cm.). It is claimed that this gives a deeper effect than the other methods.

Physiological and Therapeutic Effects

PHYSIOLOGICAL EFFECTS. Absorption of the waves results in the production of heat in the tissues, but microwave diathermy differs from other heat treatments in the distribution of the heat. The waves penetrate more deeply than do infra-red rays, but do not pass right through the tissues in any appreciable density, as does the electric field used in short-wave diathermy. Thus the effects are deeper than those resulting from infra-red irradiation, but microwave diathermy is less suitable for the treatment of deeply placed structures than is short-wave diathermy. The effective depth of penetration of microwaves appears to be about 3 cm., so the depth of heating is intermediate between that of infra-red irradiation and short-wave diathermy. With equipment generally available it is possible to irradiate only one aspect of the body at a time.

The waves are strongly absorbed by water, so tissues with a high fluid content are heated most. There is appreciable heating of tissues which have a good blood supply, such as muscle, but less heat is produced in those with a low fluid content, such as fat. Thus the heating of the subcutaneous fat, which is a disadvantage of short-wave diathermy applied by the condenser field method, is avoided.

The effects produced by microwave diathermy are those of local rise in temperature, which have been described in the chapters on short-wave diathermy and infra-red irradiation.

THERAPEUTIC EFFECTS. As the physiological effects of microwave diathermy are similar to those of short-wave diathermy, it can be used in the treatment of the same types of condition. Thus it can be used for traumatic and inflammatory lesions, in which the increase in blood supply and relief of pain and muscle spasm are of value. Also for bacterial infections, where the increase in blood supply brings more white blood cells and antibodies to the area and so reinforces the body's normal defence mechanism.

Microwave diathermy is most likely to be effective for lesions situated in the regions where the microwaves produce heat, that is in the superficial tissues and those of high fluid content. It is suitable for the treatment of traumatic and rheumatic conditions affecting the soft tissues and small superficial joints, also for superficial infections such as septic fingers, boils, carbuncles and other superficial abscesses. As it is generally possible to irradiate only one aspect of the body at a time, it is more satisfactory for localised than for widespread conditions. The ease of application may make microwave diathermy preferable to short-wave diathermy in those conditions where the depth and extent of the heating are adequate, but it is not suitable for deep or extensive lesions.

Dangers and Contraindications

BURNS. In common with other heat treatments, microwave diathermy can produce heat burns. The patient's sensation is the primary guide to the intensity of treatment to apply, so it is unwise to use the method if skin sensation is defective. Some authorities claim that the heating of the underlying tissues is greater than that of the skin, but damage should not occur if the dose is limited to that suggested.

Water is heated rapidly by the waves, so the skin must be dry and wet dressings and adhesive tape should be avoided, also areas which perspire freely. Concentration of the waves may cause overheating on application over bony prominences or in other cases where the emitter is unevenly spaced from the tissues. The effects of metal on the distribution of waves have not been fully investigated but, as with short-wave diathermy, metal objects should be removed from the field or avoided.

EYES. In animals, opacities of the lens have developed following exposure of the eye to microwaves. Consequently the treatment of eye conditions is unwise and irradiation of the eyes on the course of other treatments must be avoided.

CIRCULATORY DEFECTS. As with other heat treatments, ischaemic areas should not be treated, because of the increased demand for oxygen which results from the rise in temperature. Danger of haemorrhage, thrombosis, phlebitis and other vascular lesions also contraindicate treatment.

OTHER CONTRAINDICATIONS. Microwaves should not be applied to regions where there are malignant growths, or tubercular infections, nor to areas which have recently been exposed to therapeutic doses of X-rays. It is wise to avoid areas where the skin has been rendered hypersensitive by the use of liniments and it is said to be advisable to avoid irradiation of the testicle.

APPARATUS. Damage to the magnetron can result from leaving the apparatus on with the emitter facing a metal plate, from which the waves would be reflected. Effects on electronic devices such as cardiac pacemakers and hearing aids have not been clarified, but presumably the situation is the same as with short-wave diathermy.

Technique of Application

PREPARATION OF APPARATUS. The selected emitter is connected to the machine by the appropriate cable and the power switched on. There will be some delay before output is obtained, but then the physiotherapist tests the apparatus by placing her hand or arm in front of the emitter and increasing the output until a sensation of warmth is experienced. Controls are returned to zero and the switch turned to the stand-by position. If no stand-by switch is provided the current is turned off.

PREPARATION OF THE PATIENT. This is similar to the preparation for the application of short-wave diathermy and the reasons for each point, which are given in Chapter 20, are the same. Clothing must be removed from the area and the skin examined and dried if necessary. Sensation to heat and cold is tested at the first attendance. The patient must be advised of the nature of the treatment and warned to report immediately any undue sensation of heat or other discomfort, and of the danger of burns. He must be warned to avoid movement once the emitter has been arranged in position, and full support in a comfortable position is necessary to ensure this.

APPLICATION OF THE EMITTER. The emitter is arranged so that its surface is parallel to the skin and at the appropriate distance, due consideration being given to the surface marking of the structure to be treated. Irregular surfaces and areas which perspire freely should, if possible, be avoided.

IRRADIATION. The patient is reminded of the sensation to be expected and of the need to report accurately on that experienced. The output is then increased slowly until a sensation of warmth is experienced, or until the selected output is reached, whichever is the less. Irradiation continues for an appropriate time, the physiotherapist visiting the patient frequently to ensure that nothing untoward has occurred. The output is then reduced and switched off. Slight erythema may be observed, but there should be no marked skin reaction.

Dosage

The dose can be assessed by the power output from the machine, which is usually up to the region of 200 watts, but in all cases the sensation experienced by the patient must be the primary guide. This should never be more than a comfortable warmth and as a general rule weaker doses should be used for acute than for chronic conditions. The duration of irradiation ranges between 10 and 30 minutes, the shorter exposures being used on small areas and in acute conditions. It is advisable to commence cautiously and in all cases progression must be made in accordance to the patient's reaction. Treatment may be given daily or on alternate days.

INDEX

Printed in Great Britain for Baillière Tindall and Cassell Ltd., by
Billing and Sons Limited, Guildford and London